About the Author

I am disabled, but I do my best to remain active through writing. I refuse to give in to my illnesses. On some days, my illnesses prevent me from doing anything productive. I count a day as being successful if I can manage to put in at least one full hour of productive activity. I know that the more I accomplish on any given day, the more it will negatively affect what I will be able to do on the following day. Writing this book took several months longer than I had anticipated.

I plug away as best as I can. I write mostly about the economy. In the past I spent a lot of time helping students learn about basic economics. When direct communications with students from all over the globe became too difficult for me, I created a web site which is free for students:

www.economicsonlinetutor.com

The website is for basic concepts in economics. For discussions of economic policy and current events relating to the economy, I created a companion Facebook page:

Economics Online Tutor

I began to write essays on economics, including my viewpoints on policy. At first, I created a second section of my website for these essays. Later, I created a blog for my essays:

Jerry Wyant's Voice of Reason

I turned the text of my website into a handbook of basic economics:

"Basic Economics for Students and Non-Students Alike", by Jerry Wyant

This book can be purchased through most online book outlets. I made it available for FREE in eBook formats.

I published a collection of my essays on the economy in another book:

"Sanity and Public Policy: Separating Truth from Truisms", by Jerry Wyant

Through my essays, I was asked to join the writing staff of The Blue Route Blog. This required no extra effort on my part. I simply post on this blog what I would have posted on my own blog. The Blue Route Blog is at:

http://www.blue-route.org/blog/

The Blue Route also has a Facebook page.

I created the Making Education Work Facebook page for advocates of teachers and public education. I have written some essays for this page, and I published a collection of essays and other works in a book:

"Making Education Work", by Jerry Wyant

You can follow me on Twitter @jawyant

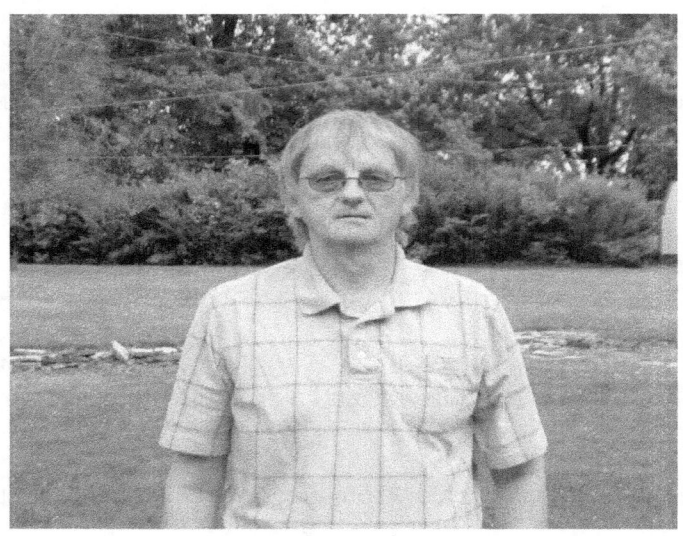

Even Great Doctors Make Mistakes

By Jerry Wyant

Table of Contents

Introduction

If I had the power, I would require every doctor to read this book. But it isn't just about doctors. I believe that I have something important to say to everybody who works in the healthcare industry. So, while I want to make sure that all doctors understand the points I am trying to make, this book is for nurses, technicians, receptionists, and other medical professionals as well as doctors.

Perhaps even more than medical professionals, this book is for medical patients. There are lessons to be learned, warnings to heed. I consider myself to be a "typical" patient. Some patients have more experience dealing with healthcare issues than I do; some patients have less experience. Some patients have more knowledge of healthcare than I do; some patients have less knowledge than I do. My "authority" for writing this book comes from my status as a "typical" patient, not from the possession of any superior knowledge. I want readers to see the typical-patient point of view. While some medical patients have more experience dealing with the medical profession than I do, and have suffered from worse medical conditions than I have, I believe that I have more experience than average. My experience provides me with several different anecdotes to use as illustrations of specific points I am trying to make.

For some time now, I have considered writing an essay or a blog post based on my personal experiences with the medical profession. I wanted to write about this subject to convey a simple message to other patients. My message to patients is this: many of our doctors provide absolutely splendid care, and we should all be lucky enough to trust that the ones we have are great doctors. But this trust should not be total or blind. Doctors are human, and even the greatest of them are going to make mistakes. We should trust them to do their jobs, yet at the same time we need to be vigilant.

Nobody is perfect, and we leave ourselves vulnerable when we have so much faith in any individual doctor that we assume he or she will never make a mistake. We are blessed to have great doctors. Even great doctors make mistakes. This simple message that I am trying to convey became the title of this book.

My story involves more than just doctors, and more than just medical mistakes. Too many patients have horror stories to tell about their dealings with the medical profession. Too many patients come away from an experience with the healthcare system feeling frustrated and thinking "they could have found a better way to handle that situation". Whoever "they" are; whether the situation is a "mistake" or whether the patient had been treated with disrespect. As a practical matter, from a patient's point of view, it isn't always easy to distinguish among a mistake by a doctor; a mistake by somebody else in the medical profession; an unnecessary inconvenience placed on patients by a facility's policies or by the healthcare system in general; and a simple miscommunication.

Because of this vagueness, and because I am speaking from a patient's point of view, many of the stories included here involve problems that cannot be classified simply as mistakes by doctors. I'm trying to address the feelings of frustrations that patients experience through dealings with people in the healthcare industry. Some of these stories include actual or suspected "mistakes" by doctors, but several of the stories obviously are not about doctor mistakes. However, these are problems that I feel need to be addressed by doctors and other professionals within the healthcare industry.

So my original idea of writing in order to send a message to patients has been expanded to also send a message to healthcare professionals. The message is this: Patients are real people, with real feelings. Patients who come to you already have problems and worries, or they wouldn't be there. They may be in pain. They may be in distress. Here are some real and personal examples of how they may feel as a result of their interactions with you, the professionals. You have the power - and I would suggest, the responsibility - to avoid letting your words and actions unnecessarily add to the worries of your patients.

I abandoned the idea of simply writing an essay or a blog post after I began writing a draft of my story. I realized that I couldn't tell my story within the framework of a normal-length blog post. I chose to write a book in which I could tell the story in a manner that I can be comfortable with, instead of writing an essay that I would feel compelled to edit heavily for length. Plus, I believe the people I am trying to reach with my message would be more likely to read a book than an extra-long essay.

The stories in this book are stories from my personal experiences. I have not gathered the stories of different people in order to make a point. This is not based on any kind of survey to find common stories. This is my story. It is the story of one patient. It is completely anecdotal and unscientific. It is not based on any superior knowledge of healthcare. It involves the people and facilities that I have personal experiences with, and nothing else. My focus is on the lessons to be learned and not on my personal horror stories. The horror stories are here for the purpose of illustrating the points I am trying to make.

The stories may be for illustrative purposes only, but they are very real. I also believe that my stories may be representative of stories that countless other patients could tell. I am not a medical professional. I want the points of view I express here to be views from a typical medical patient. As a result, I have made no attempt to become an expert on any of the medical situations which I describe in this book. Other than to mention terminology in the paperwork I have received from my doctors, I have not researched anything for this book. I am sure that my ignorance of medicine will be clear to medical professionals who read this book. But that is how it must be if I am going to get the message across that I am writing from the point of view of a typical patient.

I want readers to understand that if I experience these things, other patients are experiencing similar things. This is important to me, because perhaps professionals in the medical industry will find some of my stories to be nothing more than misunderstandings on my part. Perhaps I am missing something, and the resulting misunderstandings are due to my own ignorance. But before medical professionals write off the points I am trying to make as resulting from my ignorance, they should understand that my ignorance is shared by patients everywhere.

I have arranged the chapters in this book according to some broad points that I am trying to make. Scattered throughout the chapters are many anecdotal stories from my personal experience. These stories are not in any particular order. Most of them touch on one or more of the broad points hinted at in the chapter titles. I organized the book in this manner in order to use my personal stories for illustrative purposes only. I didn't want my personal stories to overshadow the messages I am trying to get across. For prospective on the anecdotal stories used, I placed a summary of my medical history, in chronological order, in Appendix A. Appendix B is a continuation of Appendix A, with emphasis on my current medical conditions.

These are real stories, but I have omitted all personal names and the names of specific medical facilities. Instead of the name of a doctor, I refer to a doctor by the name of his specialty or simply "my doctor". This book is not about vilifying individuals or specific facilities. Some of the anecdotes I use in this book are written with negative connotations, while other anecdotes show the same doctors in a positive light. Some of my "horror" stories involve people I believe to be great doctors. I am trying to emphasize the incidents and any related lessons we can learn from them. Using names in this book would not serve that purpose.

Since healthcare is such a hot topic of discussion these days, I feel compelled to add one more point in the introduction to this book. What I have to say in this book has nothing to do with healthcare reform. This book is not about the Affordable Care Act or alternative healthcare proposals. This book is not political. This book is about relationships between healthcare professionals and their patients, from a patient's point of view.

Doctors Are Only Human

I have had some great doctors over the years, which is a very good thing because I have had to rely on doctors to save my life on numerous occasions. I wouldn't consider all doctors to be "great", but I consider some of my doctors to have that special something that has allowed me to trust that my life is in competent hands. Some doctors fall short of that, but they all have a talent in at least one area of their jobs that I can fully respect. At least that has been my experience. I can't speak for others, but my experience with the medical profession is extensive enough to make me believe that what I have to say here is not atypical.

Without exception, every doctor I have seen has made mistakes. Even the great ones are not perfect. I trust these people with my life, yet I have learned through personal experience that I still need to be alert, I need to be on the lookout for potential oversights, and I need to question everything that doesn't seem quite right to me. This revelation should not have surprised me, and it should not surprise you.

When you think about it, doctors are human beings. How many people do you know who have never made a mistake on the job? Doctors receive many years of education and training, but how many professions are there for which education and training will guarantee that no on-the-job mistakes will be made? I certainly cannot think of any.

On top of that, think about the amount of stress involved in a doctor's life: stress relating to a heavy workload; stress relating to the frequent need to make decisions that are life-altering or life-saving, often with little time to react to the situation; stress relating to the need to follow numerous regulations and standards from different authorities; stress relating to the need to keep up with the latest developments in the profession; stress relating to the need to deal with difficult or belligerent patients and their family members; and stress relating to the knowledge of the consequences of mistakes. Given these realities, we as patients should not expect perfection.

As patients, we need to be vigilant. We need to be understanding. For one thing, a general understanding of the potential for human error should teach us to be vigilant. We need to do what we can in order to make sure that we have full confidence in the doctors we choose. And we need to do what we can to make sure that when the doctor does make the inevitable, but hopefully rare, mistake, we are diligent enough to catch the mistake before we are victimized.

What separates the great doctors from all of the other doctors? What makes a doctor great? I would guess that most patients have a pretty good idea whether or not their own doctors are great doctors. Perhaps most patients have never actually tried to define what makes for a great doctor. Perhaps many patients simply rely on their instincts to determine which ones are the great doctors. I think we all have a sense of knowing how much we trust individual doctors who have cared for us, whether or not we can articulate the reasons behind this belief. I think that if we are being cared for by a doctor who does not have our full trust, then the first step for us as patients should be to try to determine why we lack trust in that doctor. Perhaps such introspect will reveal that our fears are not justified, and we can gain trust in that doctor; perhaps not. If we still lack trust in any of our doctors after considering the reasons why, we should attempt to replace that doctor with one we are more comfortable with.

Different patients will have different points of view on what qualities separate great doctors from all the rest, as well as different points of view on which of these qualities are most important. Here is my list, which I base on my personal experiences.

1. A doctor should be able to convey to the patient that the doctor is a master of his specialty. This is an absolute must. Any doctor who fails to do this cannot be considered a great doctor. A patient who lacks faith that a doctor is a master at what he (or she) does should look for a different doctor. A doctor needs to be able to reassure his patients, not create doubts.

2. A doctor needs to be able to communicate effectively with his patients. This is a requirement for the first item on the list - the need for doctors to be able to reassure patients rather than create doubts. But there are many different types of communication involved in a doctor/patient relationship, and there are many different means and styles of communication. Different doctors have different styles, and different patients perhaps react differently to different styles. I have found that some doctors are very good at certain types of communication but not so good at other types of communication. Effective communication is absolutely vital, but there are many different ways that a doctor can demonstrate proficiency or lack of proficiency in communication. Great doctors must be able to communicate effectively with patients, but even great doctors are likely to have areas where they can become better communicators. Many of the anecdotal examples that I use in this book involve areas where a better outcome probably would have resulted from better communication.

3. A great doctor will demonstrate sensitivity, empathy, and an ability to listen to the patient's message - and not just hear the words in the message. Doctors need to understand that patients aren't medically-trained specialists and are likely to have trouble explaining their situations. Patients are likely to have doubts about a doctor who listens to a patient but responds in a way that shows that the doctor has misinterpreted what the patient was trying to say. Patients are likely to have doubts about a doctor who shows

through words or body language that he is unsympathetic to what the patients are going through. Patients are likely to have doubts about a doctor who treats patients as inconveniences. Patients are likely to have doubts about a doctor who ignores the context leading up to the office visit and instead harps on the doctor's pet peeves. Patients should not have to fear seeing a doctor because they know that the doctor is going to be bringing up issues unrelated to the reason for the patient's visit.

4. A great doctor will demonstrate a great deal of knowledge in many different areas of healthcare, not just his own area of specialty. Any symptoms that cannot be explained within a doctor's area of specialty should not be ignored, but instead handled as clues for possible referral to a doctor with a different specialty. A great doctor will demonstrate knowledge of a patient's entire medical history, not just the areas in which the doctor happens to specialize - and be able to recognize symptoms accordingly.

5. A great doctor will not leave symptoms unexplained and undiagnosed. If there is something that has not been diagnosed, then there should be a plan for diagnosis instead of simply ignoring the symptoms. A great doctor will not give up on a patient. If a doctor determines that nothing more can be done, then the doctor should be able to assure the patient that this determination is based on sound medical reasons and a thorough diagnosis of the problem.

6. A great doctor will be able to convince a patient that it is highly unlikely for the doctor to commit a medical error while treating that patient. At the same time, a great doctor will be completely open and honest about all of the potential complications with each type of treatment.

Doctors are human, and any one of them can be "great" in some of these areas but have much room for improvement in other areas. A doctor does not have to be perfect in order to be considered "great". If perfection were the standard, they would all fail. But many of them do not fail. The ones who succeed at greatness are the ones who inspire confidence with their performance instead of creating doubt in the minds of patients.

Personal Anecdote

I see some specialists for ongoing conditions. I routinely undergo various tests and procedures, and discuss changes in symptoms with my doctors. It is not unusual for doctors in these situations to prescribe a new medication. A couple of months following one such incident, which I found no reason to question, my pharmacist asked me why I was trying to refill two prescriptions for essentially the same medication. When I took that question to the doctor who prescribed both of them, the doctor admitted that he made an error in prescribing a new medicine when I was already taking essentially the same thing. I am not knowledgeable enough about prescription medication to catch such an error. If I had not tried to renew both at the same time, and if the pharmacist had not been alert enough to catch this, I would have continued to take what amounted to double the recommended dose.

From this incident, I have learned to ask a pharmacist to review my medication list from time to time, looking for questionable combinations of medication. Doctors routinely update my medication list whenever I have an appointment, and they always provide a medication list whenever I am released following a stay in the hospital. But it is not safe to assume that my doctors will have verified that my medication list is the proper one for me. Just because they have that information in writing doesn't mean that they have reviewed it.

Personal Anecdote

Somewhere in my medical records are doctor's notes implying or stating that I have been treated for depression. Such comments are not true; I have never been treated for depression. But a primary care physician once indicated such treatment in his notes following one of my medical appointments. This has created some problems for me.

The error is the result of a sequence of events involving disability. It took several years of growing medical problems for me to admit to myself that I could no longer hold down a steady job. I had to come to terms with my limitations one problem at a time. I had to deal with the fact that at any given point in time, I had health symptoms that had not yet been properly diagnosed. I clung to the hope that any day, I could receive a diagnosis for something that would be easy to fix, something that would allow me to return to my previous capacities. Over time, I was forced to accept more and more problems as being permanently disabling.

At some point in this process, I began to consider taking steps towards filing for Social Security Disability. At first, it was a back-up plan which allowed me to acknowledge that my problems could continue to get worse and not better. Long before actually deciding to file for disability status, I mentioned to my primary care physician that doing so was a possibility. I knew that his opinion would be part of the process. I also assumed that someone in his position would have experience dealing with people in my situation, and could offer me some advice.

I broached the subject, and then the doctor and I had a nice conversation about it. At the time, this was all speculation, something to plan ahead for in case my health continued to deteriorate. I had several symptoms that had yet to be diagnosed, and I would need to know a lot more about the nature of those problems. This meant more tests, which I was going to have to undergo anyway. I was only making sure I had a plan in place for my life in case these tests confirmed some of my worst fears.

The doctor mentioned what it could mean for my mental health if I could no longer work. He stated that some people can't handle the transition very well, and end up in a state of depression. He then asked me a few questions about my personal life. He said that he based these questions on his experiences with other patients. At the end of the questions, he stated that there was nothing in my answers to indicate that I was a prime candidate for depression in case I became permanently disabled. It's important to note that there was no indication at all that I had already suffered from depression. We were both speculating about what might happen in an unknown future.

That was the only time that the subject of depression came up between me and any doctor, until years later when this same doctor brought up the subject again. During an unrelated office visit, the doctor asked me how I was coming along with my depression. I thought it was a strange question, because I had visited this doctor on numerous occasions in relation to my physical health. I thought he knew my situation very well. Why would he suddenly think that I was suffering from depression? He told me that he asked the question because he looked over his own notes from my previous sessions with him and the notes indicated that he had treated me for depression.

Apparently, the doctor had wanted to make sure his notes for that day included the things we had discussed. I haven't actually seen the notes, but he must have worded them in such a way that anybody who reads them in the future, including himself, would come away with the impression that he was treating me for depression.

When the doctor used his notes from years earlier to assume that I had been seen by him for depression, he wasn't the first one who had drawn the same mistaken conclusion from the notes. At some point in time I finally decided to file for disability with the Social Security Administration. As part of the process, I had to give written permission for the doctor to turn over his notes to Social Security investigators. The process of going through a disability determination for Social Security is lengthy and complicated. A lot of information goes back and forth, and additional medical visits and tests are sometimes required. In one interim decision, I was told that my application would be rejected if I didn't visit a psychiatrist of their choosing. The reason for this determination was that my medical records indicated that I had been treated for depression but the same records didn't indicate the current status of that treatment.

I was told which doctor had indicated the treatment for depression. I knew this long before the doctor himself inadvertently told me the same thing when he asked me about my depression. But at the time that I heard this from the Social Security Administration, I assumed that this was one of their many false conclusions about my medical history. Anybody who has gone through this process with Social Security would probably know about their propensity to draw false conclusions, especially in the initial stages of an application.

I had to drive over 200 miles and into a different state in order to visit the psychiatrist who was working with Social Security on my case. The psychiatrist asked me a lot of personal questions, and then concluded that I was mentally stable with no signs of depression. I knew that all along, and Social Security would have never had a reason to question it if not for the doctor's notes.

Personal Anecdote

I had two broken arms. I had landed on my wrists during a pick-up basketball game on an asphalt surface, and the impact of landing fractured the funny bones in both elbows. I was being treated by a bone specialist in a very busy office. I was among what seemed like dozens of patients all lined up. The doctor would go down the line, take one look at a patient, give a quick diagnosis of the patient's progress based on what he saw, and then move on to the next patient. The time spent with each patient was only a few seconds. This is the way it was for all of my follow-up appointments. In my mind, it seemed like we patients were being herded like cattle.

I was told that because of my broken arms, I would not be able to work for 14 weeks. But after a few weeks, I was desperate to get back to work. I was miserable at home, and my boss kept telling me that I was needed at work. There were some things going on with new trainees that I could get under control. The issue was the use of my arms. Because I was an accountant, the biggest problem was that my job required me to lift ledgers. Other than that, I wouldn't have any problems with pens, staplers, and other office supplies. My boss joked that if I came back to work, she would simply hire somebody whose job would be to lift my ledgers for me. It was a joke, but it meant that I was wanted at work. I also wanted to be at work, and accommodations could be made for my physical limitations. So on one follow-up doctor visit, when the doctor got to my place in line, I quickly requested a release to return to work. Just as quickly, he said "Yes, I'll even give you permission to play tennis if you want." He didn't ask me whether the job requirements would get in the way of my recovery. He didn't give me an update on my healing progress since my previous appointment, even though I had noticed little change since he had told me that I couldn't return to work for several more weeks. He simply responded positively to my request and released me to return to work.

I can't say for sure that this is all good, or all bad. I knew that I could handle the return to work. As it turned out, the return to work did not create any physical problems that I am aware of. From my perspective, this was the right thing for me to do. But I question the process and the mindset of a doctor who would reverse his prognosis on the basis of my request, without any other new information. It seems to me that, at the very least, he should have grilled me on my job duties and discussed the pros and cons based on my condition.

The Face of the Facility

When dealing with patients, you are the face of the facility. Doctors, nurses, medical technicians, and others fall into this category. Receptionists are likely the first employees that patients see and talk to. Receptionists are the face of the facility throughout the check-in process and the entire time the patients spend in the waiting room. When you are in the capacity as the face of the facility, you should keep a few things in mind. Your job is a public job. Your public is there because they are dealing with problems. Many of them are in pain. Many of them are worried about things going on in their lives. They may be traumatized. They are not getting paid to be in your presence, and they are not there because they enjoy being there. They do not need you to add to their inconvenience. At the end of the day, they might not remember if you were well-dressed or well-groomed. But they will remember how you interacted with them. They will remember if they had to wait in line while you discussed personal matters or gossip with co-workers or somebody on the phone. They will remember if you spoke rudely to them. They will remember if your body language indicated that you thought of them as inconveniences. They will remember if they heard you bad-mouthing co-workers or other patients. They will remember if they had to wait, or be inconvenienced in any way, without an explanation and an apology stated in a sincere and pleasant manner.

Personal Anecdote

I showed up an hour early for my scheduled appointment. I had nowhere else to go, so I decided to wait in the waiting room. As a convenience, I announced who I was and why I was early. I figured that this would give the receptionist an opportunity to check me in at her convenience, and perhaps at the convenience of other staff members who would be involved with my care that day. Besides, there was a chance that I could get started early, which would be a convenience for me as well as the entire medical staff. I understand how circumstances throughout the day might cause medical facilities to fall behind schedule, and a convenient opportunity to get an appointment out of the way early can help alleviate the backlog later in the day.

When I announced my early presence, the receptionist greeted me with a nasty glare. "You aren't supposed to be here now", she said loudly and rudely. She then told me to go away and not come back until fifteen minutes prior to my scheduled appointment. I explained that I had nowhere else to go, and that I would like to stay in the waiting room. I was allowed to stay, but I was treated as an inconvenience just by being there. By the way, the waiting room was not crowded at that time, and there were no patients lined up to check in.

A nurse who had been scheduled to be involved with processing me as a patient was one of several people who couldn't help but overhear what the receptionist said to me. The nurse came up to me in the waiting room, quietly and politely introduced herself as my nurse, and told me that she could go ahead and begin the check-in process. I followed her around the corner, away from the reception desk, where the nurse checked me in. I ended up getting in for my procedure early.

I can add some background to help put this incident in perspective. I had gone about three-and-a-half years with a serious yet undiagnosed illness. This would turn out to be the day that the illness would finally be diagnosed properly. But it required multiple procedures, which were scheduled for the same day. First, I had to undergo some testing in the radiology department. Then, I had to go to gastroenterology for both upper and lower (GI) scopes. The combined results from these procedures would give me the long-sought answers to the questions regarding the nature of my illness. The gastroenterology department was the place where I was confronted by the rude receptionist.

I had to have these procedures at a location which is more than an hour's drive from where I live. The doctor knew I would have to come in from out of town, and this fact is one of the reasons he decided to schedule all of the procedures on the same day. My instructions were to go to radiology, and when I was finished in radiology I could go to gastroenterology. I always try to give myself extra time to make the trip from home, just to make sure I get there in time.

I showed up early at radiology. No problem - they got me right in, and I was finished earlier than anticipated. That gave me some extra time before my appointment at gastroenterology. I needed to have a designated driver to take me home following my procedures, and my driver had some local errands to run. So we left the clinic building to run these errands. I had to be fasting for my scheduled scopes, so going out to eat between appointments was out of the question. But we did take time to run errands at a few local businesses. When we were finished with the errands, we still managed to get back to gastroenterology about an hour ahead of my scheduled appointment. That is when I was so rudely greeted by the receptionist.

Personal Anecdote

I was being prepped for an angiogram and stent implant for a closed artery in my leg. I had the same procedure performed five years earlier, by the same doctor. This preparation includes a waiting time which seems like an eternity. After the IV is hooked up, it takes time before I am ready for the procedure. Also, I have to wait for the doctor to become available. The first time I went through this process, I had an additional wait because the doctor had been called for emergency surgery.

During one such waiting period, I asked to use the restroom. I might have to wait hours, and I needed to urinate before the procedure. The attending nurse refused to let me use the restroom. She insisted that I couldn't go to the restroom because the IV was already hooked up. I didn't understand what she was talking about, because I have used restrooms with IV hookups on several occasions. Instead, she insisted on inserting a catheter. She made this decision on her own and without consulting a doctor or her supervisor. She didn't even give me a choice, and I would have said no if I was offered a choice. Once I mentioned that I would need to use the restroom, my choice was made for me. A catheter in that situation defeated its own purpose. Catheters give me a constant, uncomfortable sense that I need to urinate. My point in asking to use the restroom was to avoid having that feeling for the next few hours. Instead, she guaranteed that I would.

The angiogram and stent implant process is an outpatient procedure. But there is no guarantee that the patient can go home following the procedure. It is always possible for something to happen in the operating room that will require admittance to the hospital. As luck would have it, this time I did get admitted to the hospital due to the nature of the procedure.

I was still groggy from the medication when I was sent to a hospital room. I barely remember anything that happened during or after the procedure. I was sent to a hospital room to spend the night, and I still had the catheter in place. I no longer had a need for a catheter, and I was extremely uncomfortable with it. I asked the floor nurse to remove it for me. I was told that I didn't have such a catheter to remove, because it wasn't listed on my chart. When I proved that I did indeed have one, the nurse still refused to remove it. The catheter would remain, I was told, until the doctor who ordered it sent up a different order to remove it. I explained that there was no doctor who ordered it, that a nurse from a different area of the hospital inserted it without consulting a doctor. I was then told that it wouldn't be removed until I discussed the situation with my attending physician. But the attending physician wouldn't be around until about noon the next day, when I was scheduled to be released from the hospital.

I was in a lot of discomfort because of this catheter. I wasn't willing to wait until the middle of the next day to remove something that shouldn't have been there in the first place – something that there wasn't even a record of. I insisted that the nurse do something right away to fix this problem. The nurse continued to claim a lack of authority as a reason to do nothing. I finally had to raise my voice and demanded to see the nurse's supervisor. The nurse left the room, consulted with an on-call physician, and promptly came back to remove the catheter – then apologized to me.

A Failure to Communicate

A large percentage of the situations that I bring up in this book involve a lack of communication in one way or another. The number one problem that I have seen in my dealings with the medical profession is a failure to communicate effectively. This should surprise no one. Managers and executives from all kinds of businesses will tell you that communication ranks at or near the top of the list of skills that need improvement within their organizations. I am not aware of anything about the medical profession to indicate that it would be any different. But there are many ways in which communication among patients and healthcare providers can be improved.

I have found that some doctors are much better communicators than others. The ones who are better communicators tend to have better relationships with their patients than the ones who are poor communicators.

In most cases, communication between patients and medical professionals is initiated by the patient. The patient is concerned about something, and sets up an appointment. It is up to the patient to communicate the concerns to the medical staff. The patient's statement of concern - the symptoms according to the ability of the patient to communicate them - is what tells the doctor what to look for, what kinds of questions to ask, what kinds of tests to run, and ultimately is vital for a correct diagnosis and treatment. It is up to the patient to lead the doctor in the right direction.

What should we as patients be doing in order to prevent problems caused by poor communication? How can we avoid being the source of the problem? I have my views on this subject, based entirely on what I have learned through my personal experiences. Perhaps there are other people who can come up with better suggestions than I can. I have to believe that experienced doctors and other healthcare professionals have a lot of suggestions to offer - if only they would find an effective way to communicate these suggestions to the general public.

We as patients have questions, and we need answers. That is why we visit doctors in the first place. In general, doctors in turn can provide us with answers only after we answer some questions that they have. The quality of the answers we receive from doctors - indeed the quality of the medical care we receive - depends on the quality of the information we give to our doctors and their staff. The power to avoid many unnecessary misdiagnoses lies with patients. The better we are at providing information to doctors, the better our chances of avoiding a misdiagnosis from our doctor, and the better our chances of receiving proper medical treatment.

In a doctor-patient relationship, the doctor is the professional. We need to keep this in mind in our communications. We should not visit the doctor for confirmation of our self-diagnoses. Let the doctor diagnose the situation. An attitude of "I know exactly what is wrong and what needs to be done so I'll just tell the doctor and save him the trouble of figuring it out" is misguided. You might think you are saving time, improving communication, or improving your chances of receiving proper care with this attitude, but you are not. Communication will be much better if you provide the doctor with the information he needs, by stating your symptoms and concerns and by answering his questions, instead of telling him what determination he needs to make. Let the professional do his job.

If the diagnosis is as clear-cut as you believe, then it is likely that the doctor has a systematic process for making that determination. The doctor will have sound medical reasons for using a set procedure for making a diagnosis. He will use this process even if you tell him what the answers are going to be. The patient's job is to provide whatever information is necessary for the doctor to make the diagnosis. Any other information is not useful communication. It can waste time as well as divert the doctor's concentration away from where it needs to be. If you tailor the information you give to your doctor towards a specific diagnosis, you run a risk of contributing to a misdiagnosis. Make sure you give the doctor all of your symptoms and concerns, not just the ones that you think are relevant to a particular diagnosis. Make sure you answer questions honestly concerning your symptoms, your medical history, your family history, your medication, and your lifestyle. The doctor is the professional. The doctor has reasons for wanting certain pieces of information. You are not doing yourself any favors by hiding information or by thinking "that is none of your business".

This does not mean that you always accept the doctor's diagnosis and go away quietly. As I stated above, the patient has questions, and the patient needs answers. Don't let your session with the doctor end unless you are satisfied that you have all of the answers that the doctor can give you. Perhaps the diagnosis or something else the doctor has told you has given you more questions. You are there for answers, so do what you can to make sure that you get them. Just be sure that you do not bombard the doctor with all of your questions until the doctor has given you reason to believe that he has finished providing you with unsolicited information. Doctors shouldn't be giving out answers until they satisfy themselves that they have properly diagnosed the situation, and you shouldn't expect them to.

Keep in mind that some doctors are better at certain types of communication than other doctors. I have had doctors who are very good at diagnosing problems, performing tests and procedures, and developing treatment plans – yet they were very poor at communicating to me as a patient the things that I need to know. You may have a doctor who is otherwise a very good doctor but you have to pry information out of him.

A concerned and diligent patient can get answers to questions without creating a hostile environment. There is no need to approach a doctor visit with an attitude of "by golly, the doctor is going to tell me what I need to hear, and I'm going to show that I demand answers so that he won't think I am a pushover". That kind of attitude will not only create a hostile environment, it also will likely interfere with the process that the doctor needs to use in order to provide the right answers.

Ultimately, the patients are the ones who need to ensure that proper communication is taking place. Patients are the ones whose lives are at stake. Patients are the ones who directly benefit from proper communication. Patients are the ones with questions and concerns about their own lives. The responsibility for proper communication ultimately lies with the patient.

But what responsibilities for communication lie with doctors and other healthcare professionals? They have to understand that patients are not professionals. Patients do not go through years of education and training in order to become patients. There is no common background required for patients to become patients. Not all patients are trained as expert, or even competent, communicators. A wide range of communication and language skills can be found among patients. Different people are knowledgeable in different areas, and there is no reason for doctors and other healthcare professionals to assume that patients are going to be knowledgeable when it comes to communicating issues with their own health. Nobody should assume that patients are going to understand medical terminology.

Doctors, and other medical professionals, are educated and trained for their jobs. Since proper communication with patients is vitally important in these jobs, everybody in society should be able to expect medical professionals to be competent in communication. They should not only be competent, but they should be able and willing to discuss important matters with patients at the communication skill level of each individual patient. They should be able to anticipate questions and concerns without waiting for the patient to properly communicate these questions and concerns. Language and terminology specific to the medical profession should not be used in communications with patients without explaining what they mean so that the patient clearly understands what is being communicated. Information that involves terminology new to a patient should be given to the patient in writing. New information involving unfamiliar terminology is easily forgotten.

I am being treated by specialists in several different areas of medicine. All of the specialists I see are employed in the same network of clinics. This means that they have instant computer access to each other's notes regarding my medical care. When I receive care from a specific doctor, I can choose which doctors will receive a report that I presume includes the doctor's notes as well as the specific type of care I have received and any test results. I suppose it can be quite tedious for busy doctors to routinely read and study these reports before each contact with a patient. Perhaps it is not practical to expect doctors to do this. My personal experience includes examples in which this information has proven invaluable in making a proper diagnosis of symptoms and even prevented incorrect treatment. In some cases, doctors have made a decision to refer to these notes in order to find clues regarding my symptoms. In some cases, doctors have referred to these notes only after I mentioned a prior communication with another doctor on a related matter. In some cases, doctors have asked me what other doctors have told me instead of looking in the computer to get this information directly from the doctor in question. In some cases, doctors have looked at the notes, and then asked me for clarification of something in the notes.

There also have been cases where one doctor asked me to tell him what another doctor's opinion is regarding a medical situation.

With modern technology, I see no reason why patients should be used as middle-men in communications between doctors. If a decision regarding treatment hinges on something that one doctor can tell another doctor, then it should be standard practice for the doctors to communicate directly with each other; not through the patient. If such communication is set up properly, it could even save the time and cost of additional office visits by the patient.

For their part, medical professionals - including doctors - need to understand what patients go through. I would guess that nearly everyone has had some unsatisfactory experiences with the medical profession; experiences that could have been avoided with better communication.

I guess the point I want to emphasize is that regardless of the situation or the abilities of the people involved, there is always room for improvement when it comes to communication. There is no valid reason for anybody to become complacent because they believe they already are competent communicators.

Proper communication is a valuable key to life and livelihood, and in terms of healthcare it can be the key to survival.

Personal Anecdote

I was all prepped, waiting for the vascular surgeon to perform an angiogram for my leg pain, when my blood tests came back. I had acute anemia and would not be allowed to have the scheduled procedure. My hemoglobin count was at 5.5 due to blood loss. I was told that I must have been feeling very weak with a count so low. But because of my other medical problems, I didn't feel noticeably weaker due to blood loss.

This anemia was certainly taken seriously by the hospital staff. I was told that I could not go home. I was told that I couldn't even stand up on my own. I was immediately placed in a wheelchair and taken to the emergency room. After some tests in the emergency room, I was given my own hospital room. I became an in-patient instead of undergoing the out-patient procedure that I had come in for.

While I was in the hospital, I underwent a blood transfusion. Once my blood count reached a "safe" level, they scheduled a colonoscopy for the purpose of finding a source for the blood loss. I had undergone several colonoscopies prior to this, all through the same doctor, but this time a different doctor performed the procedure. The doctors take turns being on call at this hospital, and my regular gastroenterologist wasn't on call at this time. The doctor who was on call worked through the same medical office as my regular doctor.

When I regained consciousness following the colonoscopy, I was naturally concerned about the results. I needed to know what they found out about the cause of my bleeding. This was potentially life-threatening or life-changing. It would make a difference on what I would need to do as a follow-up to the diagnosis. More immediately, I wanted to know if I could be discharged from the hospital so that I could go home.

I woke up from the procedure with the doctor and a nurse in the recovery room with me. I had a piece of paper in my hand. I looked at the paper, and it was a prescription for an enema kit. I had never had an enema prescribed for my condition, and the subject of enemas had never come up in any discussion of my condition. So now I had more questions. Why was I given a prescription for an enema kit? How would I use it?

I asked the doctor what he found out about my bleeding. I asked the doctor what the prescription was all about. He actually refused to answer any of my questions! He said that he had already explained it to me, and he was not going to repeat what he had already told me. Obviously, he had explained things to me before I fully regained consciousness. He might have thought I was awake at the time, but I remembered nothing at all. Why didn't he understand that I was asking because I didn't remember his explanations while I had been sedated?

When the doctor left the room, I asked the nurse to explain it to me. She also refused to tell me anything, saying that she didn't want to defy the doctor. I was left completely in the dark. After I was taken back to my hospital room, I asked the floor nurse if she could find out anything for me. She had some notes that did not answer my questions. When I was discharged from the hospital, my discharge papers did not have enough information to answer my questions.

After I went home, I called my regular doctor, knowing he worked in the same office as the doctor who refused to give me the necessary information. I got the answers that I needed from my doctor. But I had to wait until after I went home, and I had to make the effort to get the information from a third party.

Personal Anecdote

I had been assigned home care nursing to help me with my recovery after being released from the hospital. I had been hospitalized for complications from colon surgery. My hospital stay was for nine days, and much of this time in the hospital was because I wasn't getting enough nutrition. This was less than one month following a reverse colostomy, and I had developed an abdominal infection. Eating was very difficult for me. I would get full after a couple of bites, and I would get physically sick if I tried to eat more than that. My doctor refused to release me from the hospital until my protein and calorie intake improved to a specified level.

The doctor pushed me very hard to improve my food intake. He was stern. He kept riding me so that I would make progress every day. My intake was monitored, and there was a chart on the door to my room for the nurses to write down my protein and calorie intake. When my doctor made his rounds, he would always push me to do better. He made it abundantly clear that my job was to reach a specified level according to the food intake chart on the door. He kept insisting that I could do better. My reward for passing this test was that I would be able to go home. This gave me a strong incentive to push myself to do better.

I was being pushed, but I was given plenty of help. The kinds of food which worked best in terms of helping me reach my goal were the same kinds of food which I normally like best. My prescription was for junk food, and as much of it as I could handle. My favorite food – eggs, sausage, potatoes, and toast – was an especially good meal for helping me reach my goal. I was allowed to order food from the hospital cafeteria instead of the hospital food that is usually on the diets of patients. The doctor encouraged my visitors to bring me fast food from the outside. Doctors making the rounds - not just my attending physician but other doctors who worked the floor I was on – would bring me candy bars to snack on between meals. Doctors would make sure that the floor nurses kept bottles of Ensure stocked for me at all times.

I finally passed the test when I was able to finish my favorite breakfast. After nine days in the hospital, I could finally go home. But I was asked to have a home care nurse visit me each day, so that my intake could be monitored. Plus, I had a drainage tube for the abdominal infection, and the nurse could make sure that I was using it correctly as well as documenting the output from it correctly.

The home nurse did not work for the doctor. She didn't know the doctor, she never spoke to the doctor, and they didn't even work out of the same city. She was given instructions through the doctor's office regarding what she was supposed to do for me. But the nurse I got had her own ideas. While the doctor continued to be satisfied with my progress, she contradicted him. Through my recent experiences in the hospital, I had developed eating habits which served my progress well. I got praise from my doctor for my progress, but not from the nurse. She had her own set of nutrition statistics which "proved" that I couldn't survive if I continued to progress the way that I was going. I monitored everything I ate, and when I made progress that I was proud of, she would yell at me that it wasn't close to being good enough. She yelled at me for things my doctor was praising me for. She told me that I was going to die any day because her statistics on nutrition told her so.

I called the company she worked for to complain, and I was able to get a different nurse. The bottom line is that in situations where a patient is under a doctor's care, home nurses should not be allowed to go rogue. They should not openly contradict the doctor. They should not be yelling at, or talking down to, patients who are following the doctor's orders. If they see something that causes them to think that the doctor's orders are wrong, then they should deal directly with the doctor instead of insisting that the patient ignore the doctor.

By the way, when I entered the hospital with this problem, I weighed only 95 pounds and I had a severe abdominal infection stemming from recent colon surgeries. At the same time that I was fighting to improve my food intake, I was undergoing several outpatient procedures relating to draining the infection. I now weigh 190 pounds, and I have been told by another specialist that my rapid weight gain is responsible for increased problems associated with acid reflux. He also thinks that my ideal weight would be 170 pounds or less. In other words, according to this specialist, I gained too much weight too quickly.

Sensitivity

Different people have different prominent personality traits. Different people have different styles and methods which they tend to use when dealing with others. Different people have different approaches that seem to come naturally for them.

Different people respond differently to different approaches. Doctors and other healthcare providers should keep that in mind. And patients should keep this in mind: It isn't necessarily a bad thing if you are dealing with a healthcare worker whose overall approach is not an approach that you are comfortable with. For example, if your doctor tends to be gruff, but you are only comfortable with gentle treatment, that by itself is not necessarily a bad thing. You could be in a situation that calls for a gruff approach.

It depends on the situation. It is natural for different people with different over-riding personality traits to interact with each other. We couldn't get along as a society if we couldn't interact with those who are different from us. However, everybody could benefit by better understanding that sometimes we face situations which call for approaches other than our most prominent ones. Sometimes, a gruff doctor needs to demonstrate, to the patient's satisfaction and not the doctor's own satisfaction, that he can be sensitive. Sometimes, a doctor with an approach that is predominantly sensitive needs to let the patient know that he can be gruff.

For some of us, it is only natural to say what we are thinking. Speaking one's mind is an over-riding personality trait for many people. However, many situations exist in which it simply is not wise to do so. Sometimes, we regret what we have just said. Doctors and other healthcare professionals face many situations

every day in which discretion is necessary and speaking one's
mind is completely uncalled-for.

Personal Anecdote

As soon as I woke up from surgery to remove a portion of my stomach, I found myself in a room full of medical professionals as well as my family members. In this setting, in front of all these people while I was lying on a table waking up from emergency surgery, the only thing the surgeon said to me was "You are here because you have made bad lifestyle choices". He later backed off from that statement, after tests did not confirm his speculations.

Even if he had known with certainty that what he was saying was true, this was neither the time nor the place to make such a statement. What good could be accomplished through these comments at that particular place and time? There would be plenty of opportunities during my recovery for this surgeon to discuss my health, and any lifestyle changes I would need to make.

But he didn't know with certainty. His comments were based entirely on speculation. Later, after I had spent two weeks in the hospital, recovering and undergoing numerous tests because of complications which developed, he never mentioned any particular lifestyle as being the cause of my bleeding ulcers. There was mention of a prescription drug that had been prescribed shortly before the bleeding episode. There were numerous unanswered questions about complications which had developed. At the time that the surgeon released me into the care of a primary care physician, he did offer advice on lifestyle choices during my recovery. But he never again blamed me for nearly dying from bleeding ulcers.

Personal Anecdote

A great doctor can ease the minds of patients who are overly concerned about the unknown. Hope and optimism exhibited by a doctor can work wonders. Patients have concerns. When the doctor can dispel these concerns, the weight that is lifted perhaps can be the best medicine of all. In addition to eliminating stress, this can help to convince patients of the benefits of following the doctor's advice in terms of treatment and prevention.

Optimism can backfire, however, if it is used as a substitute for dealing with the reality of the situation. False optimism can have the opposite effects on patients. Optimism should always be used in the context of reality. It should not be used as an excuse to ignore reality.

I needed a colostomy - surgery to remove a section of my large intestine. According to the paperwork provided by the gastroenterologist who made the diagnosis, this was due to "stricture or narrowing probably caused by stroke in colon". As soon as I received the diagnosis, I was sent to a surgeon for consultation and to schedule the procedure.

This was going to be major surgery, and it was all new to me. I had previously had a gastrectomy for bleeding ulcers, but that was an emergency procedure performed when I was in no condition to make plans or to even understand what was going on. Now, for the first time, I was planning for major surgery.

The surgeon explained the process to me. It was to be a reversible colostomy, meaning that the colon would be detached, the "dead" section would be cut out, and then after a specified time period (at least two months), I would undergo another surgery to reattach the colon. In the meantime, I would have to rely on a colostomy bag for excrement. I would have to make an appointment prior to the first surgery so that a technician could mark the spot for the stoma, or the hole through my skin where the colostomy bag would be attached. Following this surgery, I would have home nurses visit me to make sure I was using the colostomy bag properly.

During this consultation, the surgeon displayed tremendous optimism. He told me that I would feel like a brand new person, which was a welcome thought after years of daily vomiting while tests were being performed in order to find a cause of my sickness. When I asked him what the potential problems were, what could go wrong, he gave me the standard "all surgeries have risks" answer, and cited statistics regarding survival rates. He did not mention any specific potential complications.

As it turned out, many things did go wrong. Nearly five years later, I am still suffering from complications. Of all the things that went wrong, none of them was specifically mentioned as a possibility until after each became a reality. As each complication developed, I was told "this happens all the time" and "this is easy to fix".

Some of the things that "happen all the time" are almost too horrible to think about. If these are common complications, or even known to be potential complications, why wasn't I informed of the possibilities ahead of time, especially when I specifically asked about potential problems? The "this is easy to fix" solutions have not fixed my problems, and today I have complications for which I am only treating with methods which have yet to "fix" anything – and this has been going on for years.

The complications started immediately after the colostomy. The system of using a colostomy bag to remove waste did not work properly. The solution that the surgeon came up with was to use Hegar Dilators. These instruments look similar to knitting needles, but thicker and rounded on both ends. A set of Hegar Dilators has several such instruments of different circumferences. They are to be inserted through the stoma and into the intestine, and then rotated until the offending stricture is properly dilated. It takes several of these dilators to do the job. You have to work your way from small to large dilators. The need for this procedure, I was told, was a common complication with colostomy. Yet I wasn't told this beforehand.

The dilators did not solve the problem. They were extremely painful to use. I had home nurses come to my house two to three times a day to work the dilators. I didn't have the same nurse every time; several different nurses took a shot at it. Together, they tried different methods in order to try to get them to work properly. All I got out of them was excruciating and unbearable pain. It was the most awful experience with pain that I have ever had – and I had to go through it multiple times every day. My whole body shook from the pain. I cried, and I had to bite down on a towel.

Some nurses tried being rough, prodding and poking hard and deep. Some nurses tried to be more patient, and let the dilators ease in to where they were supposed to go. Some nurses experimented with a combination of methods. Nothing worked. Nurses started to insult other nurses' methods.

The head nurse called the doctor to explain the problem. He assumed that they were doing something wrong, and then he questioned why they were doing it at all. He had assumed that the nurses were supposed to have taught me how to do this myself. With all of the pain that this procedure put me through, I was supposed to be the one who sticks these instruments into my intestine, through a hole in my abdomen, and then ream them around until enough excrement comes out. I was to do this multiple times per day, and use multiple instrument sizes each time.

From that point on, the nurses were there to watch me do this to myself, and to offer assistance. According to the doctor, there wasn't supposed to be any pain with this process after the first time or two. The doctor told me that the do-it-yourself approach was "normal". He told me lots of patients do their own without any problems. At the time he said that, I had trouble believing his statement. My experiences didn't make it seem possible.

Having me use these dilators instead of the nurses didn't solve the problems. The process still didn't get the required results. I still had all of the excruciating pain. But now there was an additional problem to deal with. It is not easy to deliberately poke metal instruments into your abdomen and ream them around inside your intestines when you know that the result is going to be excruciating pain.

The doctor didn't understand the problems I was having with this procedure until he was forced to see it for himself. Until then, he assumed that everybody was doing it incorrectly – and he said so.

During a scheduled follow-up office visit, the doctor grabbed the dilators and began performing the procedure himself. It was something that needed to be done, due to the problems I had been having, and he wanted to show me how to do it the right way. Once he started, he could see almost immediately that something was wrong. He finally knew that the procedure was not working the way it was supposed to work. The dilators wouldn't go into the stoma the way they were supposed to. Forcing them in only caused pain, and he could see that for himself. He could see how the procedure made my entire body shake, and made me cry in pain. He apologized for having to put me through all of this, and then he kept forcing the dilators until my stoma blew up like a volcano. There was excrement everywhere in his office, all over the table I was lying on, all over me, and all over him.

I could tell that he wanted to cry along with me. Not because of the mess that I made in his office, but because of the fact that something had gone terribly wrong and I was suffering because of it. He found me some clean scrubs to wear instead of my soiled clothing, and made arrangements to have me placed in the hospital. I wasn't even allowed to go home. I went directly from the doctor's office to a hospital room. The doctor's office happened to be in the same medical complex as the hospital, so they had hospital personnel transfer me to my new room. I had gone in for a scheduled appointment in a doctor's office, and ended up in the hospital.

The colostomy wasn't supposed to be reversed for at least ten more days, but arrangements were made to have this surgery earlier due to these complications. I'm not sure what exactly went wrong to cause these problems, but I had more complications following the colostomy reversal. Perhaps the complications before the reversal are related to the complications after the reversal.

Perhaps I could have been spared a lot of excruciating pain; perhaps the home care nurses wouldn't have been put into a situation where they turned on each other; perhaps the cost to me and my insurance company could have been reduced for home care services – if the doctor had listened to what the nurses were telling him, instead of assuming that they were all doing it wrong.

*

The colostomy and its reversal took place nearly five years ago, and I still suffer from disabling complications. These complications leave me in constant pain and affect my quality of life. But I am not receiving any treatment for this, and I have no tests scheduled in order to find a cause and a cure. At the same time, I have been given no medical reason why I should have to live with this condition. It seems like my medical records don't reflect what I am going through, and no doctor has been willing to follow up on this problem.

I was hospitalized for infection following the colostomy reversal. I nearly died on that occasion. The emergency room doctor at my rural hospital had assumed that I would die at any minute, even calling in a priest who read my last rights. I was life-flighted to a hospital with more facilities (and which employed my specialists).

43

I spent time in intensive care, weighing in at only 95 pounds. I spent nine days in the hospital, gaining strength along with the ability to eat enough to sustain me. I had a Jackson Pratt Drain inserted to remove the infection. This J-P Drain system included a drain tube and an output bottle, and required me to document both input and output. It also required another round of home care nursing, along with several check-ups and procedures at the out-of-town hospital where it had been inserted. Eventually, the infection cleared and the drain was removed. But I still have complications, and they have gotten worse over time.

I suffer from constant disabling pain from a number of different parts of my body, but many of the pain sources appear to be complications relating to my colon surgeries. I have had numerous follow-ups with the surgeon over this matter. He took a look at me, and used a medical term to name what I had. (Sorry, I don't remember the name he gave me and I can't find the page from the notepad where he wrote it down. Other than that handwritten page, the name doesn't appear anywhere in the paperwork that I received from the doctor's office). He told me it was a common ailment with an easy cure. He also told me that I would be healed in a matter of days. He then gave me a list of over-the-counter medications to take, and these medications would provide the cure.

Except that they didn't provide a cure. I called him back, and he told me that the combination of medications is different for everybody, so he had me adjust the quantities. When that didn't work, I tried a different combination according to his instructions. When that didn't work, he took another look at me. He told me that whatever it was that I had the last time he saw me was healed, but now my problem was something else – again, a medical term that I don't remember. The prescription for this was a different combination of over-the-counter medication. The symptoms were the same, but the diagnosis was different. He did tell me, in his optimistic manner, that this was a common ailment with an easy fix – just like he had told me before.

Unfortunately, this didn't work either. I went through more rounds of adjustments to the quantities of the various medications, according to the doctor's instructions. I had the doctor take another look at me, and he told me to keep trying different combinations. Nothing has worked, and this has gone on for years now.

If nothing has worked, despite years of adjustments to the medication – and if there isn't even a hint of progress, some indication that the medication is helping – then I don't understand how continuing to tinker with dosage amounts will solve my problem. I discussed this with the doctor and his staff on numerous occasions, both in person and over the telephone, and the answer was always the same – the cure is just around the corner, I just have to adjust the dosage of the same medications. After more than two years of the same thing, I finally quit wasting my time by telling him that I haven't been cured yet. I already know the answer he would give me, because he has made it abundantly clear: just adjust the dosage. To this day, I am still taking these medications, and I am still adjusting the dosage – just as the doctor has advised me to do. But I haven't been calling him to inform him of the lack of progress. And there has been no progress.

All of this over complications that I had never been warned would be possibilities - and then after they occurred I was told that they were common and had easy fixes.

I made an appointment to discuss these problems with a different doctor – a gastroenterologist who recommended this surgeon in the first place. The gastroenterologist took another look at the pictures from my recent colonoscopies, and noticed that the surgical area of my large intestine had become ulcerated. This, I was told, might be the source of my problems. I was to have another scope to determine if surgery would be required. The new scope showed that the ulcers had diminished enough so that surgery would not be required. But that doesn't explain my ongoing pain, nor does it provide for any follow-up procedure to correct my problems. I feel like I am back to where I started from, but this time I have used up my options for finding a source of the problem.

I asked for a second opinion for what the surgeon had been telling me. But I was told that he was the only doctor with that specialty who was available. I would have to move to a different part of the country, go through a different network of doctors, in order to get a second opinion.

Personal Anecdote

Following the first stent implant to open an artery in my right leg, I developed a complication: foot drop. My right foot didn't want to go along with me when I walked, and I had to drag it along. The front end of the foot wouldn't lift up so that I could take normal steps. When I visited a doctor for this, the doctor got all excited and said something along the lines of "oh my God, you will get gangrene and lose your leg! Good luck, I hope a specialist can help."

I did have a lengthy rehab process, first through a neurologist, followed by the use of a leg brace and special shoes, and finally with a physical therapist. I had to strengthen the nerves in my foot, and basically learn how to walk again. But during this process, there was never any indication that anything like gangrene was imminent – or that I was in danger of losing my leg. My family and I were put through a lot of unnecessary worry because of the reaction of one general practitioner.

Statistics are Numbers, but Patients are Real People

I'm going to make a statement that I expect many doctors will disagree with, but I'm not prepared to back down from this statement:

A doctor who treats a patient "according to the book" is making a medical error if the individual circumstances indicate that something different should be done.

Even if the doctor is following standard procedures, and even if the doctor is following orders from superiors, the doctor needs to be held accountable for this type of medical error. A deliberate effort on the part of a doctor to treat a patient in a manner that is different from what the circumstances indicate is malpractice, whether or not it is done according to procedures or direct orders.

There has to be a reason why a patient's recovery is not proceeding "according to the book", and a reason why the individual circumstances would indicate something other than what the "book" says. I can think of four possibilities.

1. The treatment used was the wrong treatment in the first place.

2. The treatment or procedure was done incorrectly.

3. An undiagnosed medical condition is causing the problem.

4. The "book" is wrong.

For any of these possibilities, it would be medical malpractice to continue to proceed "according to the book". The first three of these possibilities are things that a diligent doctor should always consider instead of simply "going by the book". The variance between what is expected and what is happening should be a red flag for any doctor. The patient is a real person whose life might be at stake.

Why should the doctor be held accountable if he is given orders to proceed in a certain way? For one thing, patients tend to expect that the doctor takes the Hippocratic Oath seriously and that this oath supersedes any other orders that the doctor is required to follow. Besides that, there is the fourth possibility which I brought up in the last paragraph, the possibility that the "book" might be wrong. If the doctor knows that the treatment is wrong, he should speak up, publicly, with outrage. The patient in the current situation should be the first to know about the doctor's outrage. The patient has a right to expect that the doctor will do everything possible to correct the situation. Without such outrage, and without a clear explanation to the patient of what the doctor intends to do about it, the doctor is complicit in malpractice.

Personal Anecdote

Following surgery to remove part of my stomach, I had been released to return to work because "the book" on that particular procedure said that a patient is ready to return to work after a certain amount of time. Until that point in time, I was still under the care of the surgeon who performed that gastrectomy. At the time I was released to return to work, the surgeon also released me into the care of a primary care physician for follow-ups. The problem is that when the surgeon released me back to work, he knew that I was too sick to work. Something had prevented my recovery from proceeding "according to the book". I had developed complications of an unknown origin while I was still in the hospital. My vital signs kept fluctuating wildly, and my blood pressure tended to be dangerously low.

The surgeon even gathered together doctors from a number of different specialties in order to brainstorm my case. They came up with some possible sources of my problem, and I was transferred to various areas of the hospital for testing. Despite all attempts, these doctors never did find a source of my problems. Eventually, my vital signs stabilized enough so that I could go home. But I remained very sick.

Despite my continued sickness from an unknown source, the surgeon released me to return to work. He explained to me that he couldn't do anything else because I had already been away from work for the allotted time for that particular procedure. The book said so.

What followed was a long nightmare for me. I suffered for several years with an undiagnosed illness that is largely responsible for my current status as a permanently-disabled person.

*

I did return to work as scheduled. I lasted about an hour, and got sent home. My employer did not want to be responsible for anything that would happen at work because of my sickness. My supervisor took one look at me and told me that I couldn't work. I explained that the doctor told me I should be at work and I wanted to give it a try. The supervisor watched me very closely. I was feeling weak, and I thought I could pass out at any time. I moved very slowly. I was nauseated. At one point, I managed to sneak off to vomit. Nobody saw me do that, and I never told anybody about this vomiting episode until now. My supervisor didn't see me vomit, but she had seen enough. She took me to the company's offices for paperwork stating that they didn't want me to work because I was too sick. I had been at work for less than an hour when I was taken to the offices.

By this time, the surgeon had released me into the care of a family physician. Based on the paperwork and story from my experience with trying to return to work, I was given about thirty more days away from work. The doctor tried to make me feel guilty about taking more time off work. He kept making comments to the effect that he was doing my employer a favor, but I should be at work because "the book" said so. He also made it abundantly clear that I could never get more than those thirty days, regardless of the status of my recovery.

The medical profession was treating my problem in the context of the surgical procedure that I had recently undergone, and there is a book on that. But my problem was something entirely different, as indicated by the undiagnosed complications which developed while I was in the hospital. Unfortunately, undiagnosed illnesses do not count when it comes to telling me what I should and shouldn't be doing. There is no book on that.

*

I returned to work according to the updated schedule. I was still weak. I was still nauseated. My abdomen was extremely painful. I had stomach cramps. I vomited on occasion. I even had occasional chest pains. The various pains prevented me from being able to concentrate on my job. Between the weakness and lack of concentration, my productivity fell to a level far below my standards – or the standards of my employer. I had been on the job long enough to have been given responsibilities beyond the basic responsibilities given to new employees in my position. I couldn't handle these extra responsibilities, and my production was well below par even for basic responsibilities. It became a problem when I was counted on to do something and I could not deliver.

I began to experience stress. Some of the abdominal and chest pains would occur when I felt stress because I was being counted on to do something which I could no longer do. I believed that this could be a complication from my stomach surgery. In a desperate attempt to save my job, I requested a transfer to a different department. I hoped that by doing so, I would become a new employee without the kinds of stress that I associated with responsibilities that had been added over time.

I lasted one week in the new department. My sickness continued to get worse, and I could no longer work.

Personal Anecdote

The year was 2007. I was very sick. I couldn't sleep, but I also couldn't get out of bed except to vomit. I was just lying there, waiting for the results from my recent upper and lower GI. In the early evening, the doctor called with the bad news. I had level 4 esophagitis (Barrett's Esophagus) and other related medical conditions. The doctor used the term "free-flow reflux" to describe my situation. Acid reflux had turned my esophagus into "hamburger". The reflux was keeping me awake, and there wasn't much I could do about it. There was a surgery for this, but I was ineligible for the surgery. The surgery involved wrapping a portion of the stomach around the esophagus. I was ineligible for this surgery because I had already had too much of my stomach removed during a previous surgery. I was told that the only thing the doctor could do was to prescribe medication. I would be required to take this medication for the rest of my life. The medication wouldn't fix the problem, but it could help to reduce it and help to control the symptoms. I had to keep my head elevated during sleep.

To this day, I cannot sleep in a bed. I find the bed to be less compatible than a couch with my need to elevate my head and change sleeping positions frequently. Nearly every night, I wake up at some point, choking on acid reflux. The symptoms persist. Sometimes the medication reduces the symptoms, but other times the medication doesn't seem to help at all. I have had the medication adjusted a few times. The level of esophagus deterioration has been reduced, but cannot be eliminated completely.

This was devastating news. I had a life-changing and even life-threatening illness which I had to deal with for the rest of my life. There was no cure; only treatment of the symptoms. But guess what? The doctor who delivered the bad news had gone out of his way to personally talk with me. He had called me after normal business hours. He gave me the news as soon as he got the test results. He didn't wait for a more convenient hour, and he didn't rely on staff members to deliver the news. He was the expert on this diagnosis, and he made sure that I got the news directly from him. This allowed him to provide me with details which might have eluded another staff member. It gave me a chance to have my questions answered directly instead of being relayed to him through someone else. Even though I got bad news, I felt reassured by the fact that I got the story straight from the doctor, and that nothing was being hidden from me due to lack of knowledge on the part of the messenger.

I was impressed with the way the doctor handled this situation. When the call came in, I was too sick to answer the phone. My wife brought me my phone and told me who was on the line. I was expecting a call from a nurse during daytime hours. Instead, I got a call directly from the doctor in the evening.

I believe that this is an example of how communications between doctors and patients can work. I have learned through later incidents that this doctor doesn't communicate with patients this way only when he has bad news to deliver. He has called me at different times of day with good news. If he is too busy, he will ask a nurse or other staff member to call me. I have seen him in action while I was being prepped for scopes. In his spare moments between duties, he is either on the phone calling patients with test results or is instructing nurses to call patients. He has shown that he truly wants to keep patients informed. Perhaps it takes a certain kind of personality for a busy doctor to spend precious moments this way, but I find it to be highly effective for successful doctor/patient relationships. Perhaps there is no such thing as being too busy for a patient.

Personal Anecdote

I had a scheduled colonoscopy coming up soon. Part of the preparation for a colonoscopy is to stop taking certain medications and supplements prior to the procedure. I have to stop taking certain meds one week prior to the procedure. I can take others up to the day of the procedure, but not take them on the day of the procedure. Others, I can continue to take even on the morning of the procedure. I am always provided with a written list as part of my instructions.

This is standard practice, and I had been through the routine several times before. When the date was approaching one week ahead of the procedure, I reviewed my list. Notably absent this time around was any mention of aspirin. I take baby aspirin once a day because of my history of circulation problems. I even have to have scopes such as colonoscopies performed in the hospital, rather than at the gastroenterology center, because I have a high risk for bleeding. Aspirin compromises the safety of the procedure. Sometimes, the doctor will want me to continue taking aspirin up to the day of the procedure due to the risk factor of not taking it; sometimes the doctor will decide that my current condition allows me to be able to quit taking aspirin a week before the procedure. In this particular instance, the doctor had not provided me with instructions one way or the other.

I phoned the doctor's office for clarification. I have called this office on numerous occasions for various reasons. There is a standard procedure for phone calls. I phone, and a receptionist identifies me by name and date of birth so that she can bring up my record on the computer. She asks me for the nature of my call. Then, she will relay the message to the proper nurse, who will return my call whenever she becomes available. I discuss the situation with the nurse. Sometimes she can answer my question directly. Other times she tells me she must consult with the doctor first, and either the nurse or the doctor will call me back with the answer.

This time, however, the receptionist did not follow the same procedure. When I told her the nature of my call, that I needed clarification from the doctor as to whether to stop taking aspirin a week ahead of the scheduled procedure, she did not consult anybody. The receptionist just told me to stop taking aspirin. That was her answer, and she even told me that she based it on what she believed the doctor would say if anybody bothered to ask. Well, I was asking, but the receptionist was trying to leave the doctor out of the process of answering my question. When I told her that there were other circumstances involved in my case, she did not offer to relay the information to a nurse. She made it very clear from her words that she did not want to go to the trouble of relaying my message. The receptionist expected her own answer to be the final answer to my medical question.

If I didn't have a history of knowing that the doctor has to make this decision for me on a case-by-case basis, I might have just taken her word for it. If I didn't know the office's procedures well enough to know that the receptionist wasn't the person who should be making that decision, I might have taken her word for it. I have to wonder how many patients have been given unsound medical advice because the wrong person answered the phone. In this case I knew better, so I insisted that she relay my message. It turned out that the doctor himself called me and told me that he needed more time to review my current situation before he could give me the answer. He called me back, in the evening after normal working hours, and told me that I most definitely should continue to take the aspirin. This is in direct contrast to what the receptionist tried to get me to agree to do. When the date of the colonoscopy arrived, the first thing the doctor asked me was whether his instructions to me over the phone were clear. He was genuinely concerned that I would mistakenly quit taking the aspirin.

Personal Anecdote

I had a stent implant for a closed artery in my right leg, which is an outpatient procedure. In this case it was the second time I had undergone this particular procedure. Such procedures are performed with the stipulation that if complications develop, I might be required to spend the night in the hospital for observation. In this case, that is what happened. The vascular surgeon had to use a new type of procedure, and as a precaution wanted me to spend the night in the hospital for observation.

This is something that I knew going in would be a possibility. Going in, not knowing that I would be staying overnight, I was required to have a designated driver. But when I was forced to stay overnight, my driver could not stay. She had her own business to attend to. She would have to return to pick me up when I was released. She would need to know what time to be there, because she would have to work her own schedule around picking me up. The drive time involved was more than one hour each way.

In the morning, following breakfast, I was declared ready to go home. I was already dressed. I had already signed the release papers. The doctor had told the floor nurse - over the phone - that I could go home. Except that I had to stick around until he made his rounds and visited me. I waited. I waited some more. Hours passed, and I was sitting on the hospital bed, all dressed and packed, just waiting for the doctor to show up. I was told that it could be "any minute now", but the minutes turned into hours. In the meantime, my driver was in limbo. She had her own business to take care of, back home. She couldn't afford to leave home and then wait all day for the doctor to show up. The doctor wouldn't give me a time frame, just that it would be "during his rounds", which included patients in two or three different hospitals. I knew that I would have to wait until the doctor showed up, then call my driver, and then wait over an hour for the driver to show up. And the driver's entire day was being inconvenienced.

As time passed while I waited, I was getting more and more upset. I was ready to explode. Finally, after lunch, the doctor walked in. He had deliberately made me the last stop in his rounds, but he hadn't bothered to tell anybody. He saved my stop for last because he wanted to be able to bring a cardiologist with him to write a prescription for statin drugs. Statins are for treating high cholesterol. I didn't have high cholesterol, but the doctor wanted me to take the medication because he considered me to be a high risk for developing cholesterol problems in the future. I had been waiting hours just so the doctor could bring in another doctor to write a prescription. The prescription went directly to my pharmacist anyway. I didn't need to be in attendance while the doctor wrote it. I was never told why I needed two different specialists to write one prescription.

I was still fuming when I finally got to go home. I had been rude to the doctor when he walked in. When I saw him, I asked "where have you been?" in an unpleasant manner. He looked at me like I had hurt his feelings. He said something along the lines of "I thought you would appreciate the extra effort I had to go through during your procedure." And I did appreciate his efforts and his talents. I just didn't appreciate having to wait for hours, expecting him to show up at any minute, after I had already been told that I was ready to go home. I didn't appreciate his lack of understanding the position I was in because of it, or the position my designated driver had been put in.

I wasn't rude to him after he made that comment. But I still wasn't happy about the way he handled the situation. My experiences with this doctor had already told me that he is a great doctor in terms of his talents as a surgeon. But he is not so great in terms of communicating with patients. I already knew that before this particular incident. But this incident stands out as the most glaring example.

Keeping Things in Perspective

Patients come to doctors with problems. Patients have health issues, and they see doctors for solutions to these health issues. Doctors are trained to diagnose, treat, and/or refer the patients accordingly. The doctors rely on clues based on such things as the patients' symptoms, medical histories, test results, family histories, and lifestyles. It is important for patients to provide thorough and accurate information to the doctors in order for proper treatment to ensue.

It is equally important for doctors to be able to weigh the clues objectively in order to assess their importance to the issue at hand. Doctors are trained to read symptoms and test results. They are also trained to understand the health ramifications of certain lifestyles and certain family histories. Unfortunately, some doctors fixate so much on the ramification of certain histories that they ignore, or at least downplay, other clues and even the reason the patients come to see him in the first place. Just because doctors are trained to know that certain histories or lifestyles are likely to create bad health results does not automatically mean that every patient health complaint is due to those histories and lifestyles. Other symptoms and clues should not be ignored or downplayed. Perspective is in order, and some doctors are so fixated that they lack perspective. When perspective is lost, misdiagnosis is likely.

Personal Anecdote

I have never been diagnosed with high cholesterol. My cardiologist told me that, if anything, my cholesterol level is slightly "too low". Yet due to my history of circulation problems, I have been identified as high risk. Statins were prescribed because of this risk factor. I had some side effects, though. Statins gave me headaches, something that I had never had a problem with before. I also started getting dizzy spells. I explained these side effects to the doctor. He insisted that I must take this medicine, but he did agree to cut the dosage in half, and doing so did help somewhat to decrease the side effects. I still got headaches and dizziness, but it wasn't as bad as it had been with the higher dosage. I continued to take this medication as prescribed.

While statins were prescribed due only to a risk factor, I have real problems because of complications from colon surgeries. These complications remain to this day as the sources of chronic pain and discomfort which are with me every moment of every day. Pain and discomfort prevent me from doing many things that I previously would have considered to be routine. This is most definitely a life-altering condition. It comes in multiple forms, and at any given time one form of pain and discomfort will be stronger than the others, until one of the others takes over as the overriding pain of the moment. This is an ongoing problem for me. The pain and discomfort never decrease. I have been given a smorgasbord of over-the-counter remedies. This doesn't help, so the doctor makes adjustments to the combination of medications for me to take. To this day, nothing has worked, and the pain and discomfort continue to increase. I know that this problem is a complication from my colon surgeries, but it could have a combination of sources. Perhaps the surgery to remove a portion of my stomach is also a factor. I don't know, because a specific source has not been identified. I have been diagnosed, through colonoscopies, with having ulcers in the location of the large intestine where the colon had been reattached. The colonoscopies have shown that the ulcers are decreasing, so a surgical solution has not been recommended. The ulcers may be decreasing, but the pain and discomfort are not.

Because the smorgasbord of over-the-counter medication has not reduced the problem, my surgeon took a closer look at my overall medication list. He immediately told me that I must stop taking statins because they cause some of the very same problems that I am being treated for. These problems include abdominal pain, nausea, bloating, gas, and bouts of diarrhea and constipation.

So I had one doctor treating a serious problem telling me that I cannot take statins, and another doctor telling me that I must take statins due only to a risk factor. I took a closer look at the known side effects from statins, and I found some others which are problem areas for me – drowsiness and difficulty sleeping.

It seemed obvious to me that I needed to stop taking statins. However, the doctors giving me contradictory instructions would not communicate with each other to sort this out. They insisted that I act as middle-man between them. It was up to me to tell one doctor what the other one said, relay the response, and continue to work back-and-forth between the doctors until they could agree on a solution to this disagreement.

I should note that there were three doctors involved: the surgeon who performed the colon surgeries and who was treating me for the complications; a cardiologist; and a vascular surgeon. All of these doctors work for the same healthcare organization and have access to the exact same information about my medical history. They share the same computer system, and my medical history is in that computer system. Yet they all left it up to me to act as an intermediary in communications between them regarding conflicts with my treatment. With modern technology, I don't understand why we don't have a system in place so that doctors will discuss such issues directly with each other, rather than relying on patients with no medical training to relay messages. This is not the only time in my role as a patient that I have acted as a middle-man between doctors.

The cardiologist and vascular surgeon were adamant that I needed to continue taking statins, even after I relayed to them what I had been told by my colon surgeon. They were very defensive about statins. They kept asking me "why" even after I had already explained what I knew. They demanded more information from me than a non-professional like me could give them. They acted as if their feelings were hurt by suggestions that statins have any side effects at all. I even told them that I would be willing to take frequent cholesterol tests, and as soon as the tests indicated an elevated level of bad cholesterol, I would be willing to start taking statins again. That suggestion went nowhere. I was prescribed a different kind of statin medicine as a compromise.

But that wasn't acceptable to the surgeon who had told me to stop taking statins. The problems were with statins in general, not a specific type of statin. I needed to quit taking all statins. When I relayed that information, I had to go through another round of answering the "why did the doctor tell you that" questions – again, these were questions which obviously I am not qualified to answer. After several rounds of back-and-forth messaging, including office visits and telephone calls, and involving staff members from three different clinics as well as the doctors themselves, no agreement could be reached. The doctor who prescribed the statins continued to say that I should take them, but he told me to do what I thought was best. I quit taking statins, but I am aware of the risk factor.

Personal Anecdote

My young daughter was on her way to visit me while I was in the hospital recovering from stomach surgery, and I was concerned that the oxygen tube on my face would frighten her into thinking horrible thoughts about my condition. I knew that she had been frightened in the recent past by people who were visibly sick, people who, because of medical conditions, didn't look "normal" to her. I worried that seeing me that way would make her scared of her own father. She was just a young child, after all. Since she was only going to be there about ten minutes, I asked the nurse if I could remove the oxygen for that period of time only. I explained why I was making the request. The nurse sternly said "no", and left it at that.

Perhaps there was a medical reason why I couldn't remove the oxygen for ten minutes. I was never given a reason why it had to be in place with no exceptions even for a short period of time. It would have been nice if the nurse had explained, in a friendly tone, why my request could not be granted.

Personal Anecdote

When I was finally released from the hospital following a gastrectomy and two weeks of complications, my discharge papers included instructions for me to drink plenty of fluids. I took this to mean that I needed to drink lots of water, which I did. However, during a follow-up office visit, the surgeon clarified the instruction and told me that I needed to drink Seven Up, not water. So from that point on, I made sure that I drank plenty of Seven Up every day.

After that visit with the surgeon, I was released into the care of my primary care physician. He told me that the surgeon was wrong, and that I should not be drinking Seven Up. He told me that I should drink Gatorade instead. I asked him why, and he gave me an answer which indicated that he has a general policy of recommending Gatorade to patients. His answer in no way reflected my specific condition.

I was torn between two different recommendations: one from a surgeon who had been directly involved in my care; and one from a general practitioner who hadn't been involved, but nonetheless told me that the surgeon was wrong. Based on my personal knowledge of what I had been going through, as well as verbal and non-verbal communication from both doctors, it was easier for me to trust the recommendation of the surgeon. I continued to drink Seven Up on a regular basis. However, I did keep Gatorade around to drink occasionally.

Medical Errors and Misdiagnoses

For this book, I am using only my personal experiences as illustrations for the points I am trying to make. Using only personal experiences as a guideline for this discussion, I cannot possibly address the types and frequency of medical errors throughout the healthcare system. That information is available through other sources, at least statistical versions of the information are available, and I'm sure many readers have their own horror stories to add. Since the subject of medical errors is central to my purpose for writing this book, I want to point out the medical errors and misdiagnoses from my personal experience. This is certainly not a comprehensive list of errors that patients in general can or do experience, nor is it a list of the most common errors. I am simply pointing out errors from my personal care. Besides the lessons that can be learned about each type of situation, I am trying to emphasize the lesson that these errors are personal. They involve real people. In my case, they involve me, which from my perspective makes them very personal indeed.

People make mistakes in all areas of life, but when it comes to medical care mistakes can have dire consequences for patients. There is no acceptable level of mistakes in medical care – not if I stand a chance of being a victim. I'm not the only patient who feels this way. No matter how low the percentage of medical errors, if it is greater than zero then nobody wants to be in that percentage. The point is that no healthcare personnel should be proud of a low number of errors unless that number is zero and can reasonably be expected to stay at zero. Each error has the potential to do great harm to a real human being. Statistics are numbers, but patients are real people.

Although a focus on medical errors is central to this book, most of the incidents that I use as examples cannot be classified simply as

66

medical errors. I am using my own experiences to illustrate various areas of concern regarding patient care. Some of these areas of concern clearly are not what people would consider to be in the same category as a misdiagnosis or other medical error. Some of them might involve only a miscommunication. There is a gray area surrounding many incidences when it comes to categorizing problems as medical errors. Some problems do not directly involve a wrong treatment, but perhaps could potentially contribute to a wrong treatment. Those kinds of problems can be categorized as something other than simply calling them medical errors. Some of the problems might involve only judgments which I question or which later proved to be incorrect. Some of the problems that I mention might not even be problems with my healthcare at all. Perhaps I think they are problems because I have misunderstood something. I am not an expert in healthcare, I am only a patient.

But there are some incidents which I cannot classify as anything other than medical errors. I do want to note that even though I consider medical errors to be a serious issue, and one that I take personally when they affect me, I consider some of the doctors involved in these incidents to be great doctors. I have no reservations about receiving care from them. The incidents serve to illustrate the idea that patients should be diligent even when it comes to the doctors they trust the most. Even great doctors make mistakes.

Personal Anecdote

At age 49 I had a spell that is difficult to describe, but it felt like my entire body cavity went numb. This is something unlike anything I had ever experienced before. I visited a family doctor who listened to my symptoms, then looked over the form that medical offices often make you fill out – the one that has you check off general symptoms, family history, etc. For reasons that I don't know, he focused entirely on one digestive problem that I had when I was a young child. Based on that "diagnosis", he prescribed a certain medicine. Unfortunately, I do not remember the name of the medicine. Immediately after I began to take this medicine, I nearly died from bleeding ulcers. I had never been diagnosed with ulcers before. I had emergency surgery, followed by numerous complications. At the time of dismissal from the hospital following surgery, according to normal procedure, the nurses were explaining the meds that I would need to take. Missing from the list was the one prescribed by this family doctor. When I asked if I should continue to take it, the nurses checked with my attending physician who told them something along the lines of "absolutely not, that medicine is what caused the bleeding in the first place". I do not have this in writing, but it is the only explanation for a cause of my bleeding that anybody at the hospital offered after the surgery and several tests relating to the complications.

Personal Anecdote

My physical condition deteriorated after I was released from the hospital following a reverse colostomy. Instead of the expected recovery, I kept getting sicker and sicker. I ended up in the local hospital's emergency room. This is not the same hospital which employs my specialists, and it is not the same hospital where my surgeries were performed. The local hospital is a rural hospital which is not equipped to deal with my specific problems.

Although I was drifting in and out of consciousness, I could tell that the emergency room doctor was befuddled. He paced around the floor, and kept making comments to the effect that there was nothing he could do for me. He sent for a priest, who came into the emergency room and read me my last rites. The doctor thought I was going to die, and he made no attempt to save me.

My wife kept telling him to check with my specialists, and to send me to the hospital where my specialists work. Finally, he called for an air ambulance, a life-flight helicopter, to take me there. After a helicopter ride, for which my insurance was billed over $20,000, I got the treatment that I needed in the intensive care unit. I checked in weighing 95 pounds. My problem turned out to be related to abdominal infection stemming from my recent surgeries. Recovery from this incident involved a 9-day hospital stay, a JP Drain (drainage tube inserted in my abdomen attached to a collection bottle), several out-patient procedures relating to the drain, home nursing care, and a very rough road for me in terms of being able to regain the ability to ingest enough food to sustain me.

My attending physician for this incident, once I made it to the right hospital, was the surgeon who had performed my colostomy and reverse colostomy. He did not hide the fact that he was very upset that the emergency room doctor had not consulted him. He also told me that although I was sent to the right place eventually, he believed that the $20,000 helicopter ride would have been medically unnecessary if he had been consulted.

Personal Anecdote

My current medical problems began in 2004. The first sign that something wasn't quite right was the fact that on several occasions I would turn my ankle while mowing the lawn. Any little hole or depression in the yard, and my ankle would turn in a grotesque manner. My experiences as a basketball player taught me to recognize when an ankle is in a position it shouldn't be in. I was experiencing the same thing, except without any pain or swelling.

Later, I did experience pain. But the pain wasn't associated with a turned ankle. My pain occurred from walking, and it was always in the right leg. The pain would start in the upper thigh, with a tightening sensation, and then move all the way down my leg. The pain would go away after several minutes of rest. Although I could get rid of the pain through rest, it would start up again whenever I walked.

I sought medical help, and was referred to a vascular surgeon. After some tests which indicated a closed artery in my right leg, the vascular surgeon scheduled me for an angiogram. He also gave me a very gloomy prognosis. He even drew me a picture indicating all of the arteries around my aorta which were blocked. He made this prognosis on the basis of my leg pain, the test results indicating a blocked artery in the leg, and the fact that I am a smoker.

During the angiogram, the doctor kept muttering in amazement that what he was seeing was not what he had expected. There was no widespread damage around my aorta or throughout my arteries. There was a closed artery in my right leg, but that was the only damage that he found. He placed a stent to open this artery. Then he apologized for being wrong about the diagnosis. The symptoms and test results did indicate the actual damage which was found. But he had told me there was much more damage than what was really there, and that was the basis for the gloomy prognosis. He had only speculated on the rest of the damage, basing this speculation on my smoking habit. For his diagnosis, he had let his knowledge of the potential dangers of smoking override the actual evidence in front of him.

It would have made sense if he had drawn the picture to indicate what could happen to a smoker. But that isn't what he had done. He had given me a pessimistic diagnoses based on his assumptions of what he believed had already occurred.

Balancing the Costs and Benefits of Medical Tests

How many tests are necessary? I have learned through personal experience that it would be more appropriate to ask which, not how many, tests are necessary.

Some doctors order medical tests as a matter of routine with no regard for, or understanding of, the costs involved. Sometimes, the tests are not based on expected medical benefits that are sufficient to justify the costs. This situation would not occur if doctors understood the costs involved and based the decisions to order tests on individual circumstances, instead of doing so as a matter of routine.

The same thing could be said about follow-up doctor visits and procedures. What are the costs, and are the potential benefits high enough to justify the costs?

On the other hand, sometimes individual circumstances justify follow-up visits, tests, and procedures that are not ordered. If the current treatment is not progressing as expected, then both doctor and patient should have an explanation for this situation – an explanation that is based on the true cause of the problem and not on mere speculation. There might be an underlying, undiagnosed medical problem that requires treatment. Testing for possible causes, even if the areas tested are not within the doctor's area of specialty or part of the doctor's routine pattern of ordering tests, would be justified in this case.

I have suffered from having tests and follow-ups that were unnecessary. I have suffered from not having tests that would have revealed the source of known symptoms of diagnosed origin. It works both ways.

The number of tests isn't as important as getting the reasons for the tests right in the first place.

Personal Anecdote

I was sick and getting sicker. I was suddenly unable to work. I had no answers to the source of my sickness.

This was a huge financial setback for my family. I had a vested interest in a modest retirement fund, and we were forced to use that for living expenses. I was able to switch to my wife's health insurance policy, but that policy was inferior to the one that I had when I was working. It was at this time that I decided to file for Social Security Disability benefits. But that process takes years to go through, and my application was severely hindered by the fact that many of my problems remained undiagnosed. I could explain what I was going through, and how it prevented me from working. But that didn't really matter to the SSA. Social Security doesn't recognized undiagnosed illnesses. My ability to have my disability claim approved was very much in doubt, and even if it was approved it would take years before I would know – and longer before I could receive any benefits.

I continued to seek a medical answer for my problems. I was in the care of a family physician, and he acted as if he had no clue as to how to get these answers. He did refer me to a gastroenterologist for some scopes. I have been in the care of the same gastroenterologist ever since.

The specialist was looking for something to explain my condition. He did find a severe case of Barrett's Esophagus. I am being treated and undergoing follow-up scopes for that condition. But that wasn't the source of the main problems I was experiencing at the time. Even so, I began to feel a little better while sitting at home resting. Between feeling a little better, and the financial strain on my family, I decided to attempt going back to work. But I knew that I could no longer do the same kind of work that I had done before, so I took a job with little physical and mental stress.

I became sicker and sicker as time went on. I started vomiting on a daily basis. I had to sit or lie down so that I wouldn't pass out. I got severe stomach cramps. These problems continued to get worse. I was vomiting several times a day. My stomach cramps became almost constant. I missed a lot of work until I was forced quit my job. I had picked that job because of its low physical and mental stress, and giving it up meant that I could no longer work at any regular job. I had done everything that I physically could do in order to remain employed, but none of my attempts were successful.

I was seeking a medical answer to my worsening sickness. My condition was being treated as if it had something to do with my previous stomach surgery, because that was the medical history that the doctors had to work from. When all tests and scopes failed to reveal the source of my problems, the gastroenterologist finally decided to have tests run for problems in areas other than my stomach. These tests finally revealed the source of my problems. The problem was in my colon. According to the gastroenterologist, a "stricture or narrowing probably caused by stroke in colon". That's the way he worded it for my paperwork. He explained to me that a section of my colon had died due to an undetected stroke from years earlier. He openly speculated that this stroke likely occurred while I was undergoing stomach surgery. I was sent immediately to a surgeon to schedule a colostomy.

Three-and-a-half years had passed between the time of my stomach surgery and my colostomy. During that time, I became very sick. I lost not one, but two jobs, and became permanently disabled. I underwent numerous tests in search of answers. It was only after they started looking somewhere other than my stomach for the problem did I finally get answers. Assumptions based on my recent medical history had prevented doctors from looking in the right place. Ongoing testing in the absence of a medical explanation for my problems finally gave me the answers I needed - and probably saved my life.

Personal Anecdote

Following my gastrectomy, my vital signs indicated an unknown problem that could be life-threatening. Of particular note was a very low blood pressure. A team of doctors from different specialty areas got together and decided that I should undergo many different tests for different potential sources of this problem. I was moved around to different sections of the hospital for these tests. One of them happened to be cardiology. The doctors had decided that it was possible that I had suffered a heart attack during surgery, which would explain my symptoms. I underwent extensive testing and observation, and my heart was pronounced healthy. Heart problems were ruled out as a source of my problems.

But because I had undergone the tests, a heart doctor placed me in follow-up. I became a heart patient for the simple reason that I had undergone tests. The fact that the tests were all negative didn't seem to matter. Shortly after being released from the hospital, I started receiving notices to set up a follow-up appointment with this doctor. At first I ignored the notices, knowing that this kind of appointment was unnecessary in my case. But when the doctor persisted, I relented and set up an appointment. In doing so, I was casually notified that the doctor would need current test results to go along with this appointment. So they scheduled tests for earlier in the day. This was clearly identified as being a routine procedure that the doctor required of his patients for follow-up office visits.

No medical reason was given to me for these tests. The doctor had determined that he wanted them performed as a routine procedure. There was no medical reason for me to even have an appointment; I only agreed to it because the doctor had been persistent and I wanted to get him off my back. The tests were negative, as I had expected. The doctor released me as a patient following that office visit because there was no reason for me to continue following up on a non-existent problem. But when I got the bill for the routine test, I was shocked. Neither the doctor nor I knew the cost involved.

The insurance company paid this cost. In other circumstances, I might not even have noticed how high it was. But I had just switched insurance plans and I knew that after a certain dollar amount, I would be required to pay 100% of all medical expenses until the total annual out-of-pocket amount reached a catastrophic level. This occurred in January, and that one test, the one that I didn't even need, took me directly to the point where I would be responsible for 100% of medical expenses for me and my family. I effectively lost insurance coverage for the entire year, unless I exceeded the amount required to get me to the copayment portion of my policy. I would likely be bankrupt if I got that far. I definitely took notice of this, and I was devastated.

I did some research, and I learned that the reason the cost of the test was so high was that the hospital had added a very expensive facility charge to whatever the doctor and the technicians charged. This was legal, and the insurance company did not question it, because of an agreement with rural hospitals to reimburse them for providing certain procedures. This agreement directs more patients to rural hospitals. If I had the same tests performed at an urban hospital, it would not have been very expensive at all.

My lessons from this incident:

1. Question all doctor requests for tests and even for routine office visits in order to determine if they are necessary. Don't agree to anything unless you have reason to believe they might be necessary.

2. I now refuse any tests or procedures at my local rural hospital. I insist on making my appointments at an urban hospital. I have to drive 130 miles to do this, but it is much cheaper than paying facility fees in addition to all other charges.

3. Patients at rural medical facilities are paying quite a bit more than patients at urban medical facilities for the exact same procedures. Based on my conversations with a number of doctors and nurses, I don't believe very many people are aware of this. I understand the reasons insurance companies would want to direct business to rural facilities. But if more people were aware of how much this adds to medical costs, this policy would result in less, not more, business for rural facilities.

Personal Anecdote

One of the frustrating things about my medical history is that I always seem to have symptoms of health problems which have yet to be diagnosed. I continue to be frustrated in this way.

Sometimes, a specialist will use all of the testing tools available to him and still not get an answer to my problems. This often leads to speculation that perhaps the problem is in an area that previously had not been looked at. My colon problems went undiagnosed for almost four years because doctors had assumed that my problems were directly related to my stomach surgery. Only after they had run all of the tests that they could on my stomach did they start to look elsewhere for the source of the problem.

On one occasion, I had discussed my symptoms with a gastroenterologist, who combined the information I had given him with what he already knew from my medical history, and decided that it would be a good idea if I visited an urologist. He didn't try to speculate that the urologist would find the source of my problems; he only knew that the problems lie somewhere other than where he had looked, and an urologist might be able to solve the mystery. If not, that information also would be useful for eliminating possibilities. Besides that, the gastroenterologist thought that someone my age probably should see an urologist if any symptoms are present to indicate a potential problem with my bladder or prostrate.

Except that one specialist cannot refer me to another specialist. Referrals must go through a primary care physician. When I explained to my family doctor that I would need a referral to see an urologist, he gave me a dirty look. He told me that he had just read some negative things about urology in a medical journal. He then went into a rather lengthy rant, basically saying that all urologists are quacks. He finally gave me the referral I had asked for, but only on the basis of honoring the wishes of the gastroenterologist who made the suggestion.

If he was going to give me the referral anyway, he could have done so quietly and kept his biases to himself. Or am I better off knowing what his biases are?

Personal Anecdote

I was prepped for an angiogram. This was the second attempt to find the source of increased leg pain. I already had stent implants for pain in the same leg; this latest procedure was designed to look for the source of new pain. My first attempt at this procedure was aborted at the last minute due to the discovery that I had severe anemia.

This time, I had a new concern. I had recently suffered from bouts of worrisome chest pains. The pains would last for five minutes or longer, sometimes as long as thirty minutes. The pains would be infrequent, but they seemed to be coming more often. At the time of my scheduled angiogram, I was getting these chest pains two or three times per week. After each pain passed, I would feel too weak to do anything for the rest of the day. It's difficult for me to describe, but I would have a sensation in the back of my neck – perhaps at the base of the brain. My impression was that whatever the sensation was, something had settled in my spinal cord. This was definitely something that concerned me.

I made sure to report the chest pains to the nurses when I checked in for the scheduled angiogram. The nurses notified the doctor at the same time that the staff started to wheel me towards the operating room. Fearing a heart attack, he stopped the procedure before it began. I was immediately transferred to the cardiology section of the hospital. I was already prepped for an angiogram, and they decided to have the procedure to look at my heart instead of arteries in my leg.

Speculation ran rampant between the time they decided to move me to cardiology and the time of the actual procedure. I was told that I likely had suffered a series of heart attacks. They even told me which sections of the heart had been affected, and how. I was told which medications I would need once I left the hospital. The hospital staff was alerted to prepare for open heart surgery.

The results of the procedure were quite different from the speculation. There had been no heart attack. My heart showed signs of being in excellent health. They did find a previously-undetected blockage of an artery leading from my aorta, but this had already self-corrected by creating its own natural bypass. The doctor did not believe that any corrective procedure would be required. He prescribed a beta blocker to take daily, as well as nitro pills to take during incidents of chest pain.

During a follow-up office visit with a cardiologist who had recently been assigned to me, the doctor took several minutes to review my entire medical history. All of my specialists were in the same network of clinics, and computer access to this information is readily available to all of the doctors within that network. After reading through my medical history, he stated that he didn't believe my chest pains had anything to do with my heart or with my circulation at all. He suspected that the pains were a symptom of Barrett's Esophagus, a condition for which I was already being treated. He had me go through a series of tests, including a nuclear cardiac stress test and I believe an ultrasound. The tests confirmed his speculation. My chest pains were not related to my cardio system at all, but were the result of worsening symptoms involving my digestive system.

Among other things, this meant that the treatment would be different. He explained how the chest pains would respond to the nitro pills, but nitro pills wouldn't be the most effective way to deal with these pains. The best prescription would be for me to take over-the-counter antacids. The antacids can prevent incidents of chest pains from occurring as long as I take them at the right time.

This revelation worked wonders for me. I still get occasional chest pains, and they still knock me for a loop when they occur. I still need a day or so to recover from their effects when they occur. But the incidence of chest pain is much less frequent because of this change in treatment. When the chest pains do occur, I can normally get them to end much quicker through the use of antacids rather than relying on nitro pills. Rather infrequently, the antacids don't seem to help during incidents of chest pain. I keep nitro pills around for those situations.

Questionable Billing and Unethical Practices

Let's face it. The average patient has no way of knowing the accuracy of a medical bill. The list of fees on an itemized bill often includes items that the average patient will find surprising. The number of different bills from different medical professionals, facilities, and organizations for what the patient considers to be one single, simple procedure can also surprise patients. The documents that a patient receives from their insurance company often only serve to complicate the issue with different numbers, different ways to summarize the information, even different terminology than the information from a medical bill for the same procedure. Patients can even be confused over what may appear at first glance to be a random method for the insurance companies to decide which items to pay without question and which items to delay or refuse payment on. It is futile for patients to try to figure out the difference between the amount billed by the medical facility for any given line item and the amount that the insurance company says the facility is allowed to collect for that item. The only thing that patients can know about these items is that without group insurance rates the medical facility would demand that the patients pay the full amount on their bill, not the amount that the insurance company says the item is worth.

And the dollar amounts listed? Patients have no way to understand why a certain line item costs a certain amount or why two line items which are identical in the patients' minds have different costs. I have spoken to several medical professionals, some who work in billing departments and some who are doctors and nurses, and most of them cannot identify the reasons for specific items on a bill. In many cases, the billing is an outsourced service, provided by a company other than the care provider. The only answer I get is that the item and its cost are based on codes input by clerks, and the clerks have guidelines to follow. Knowing what those guidelines are, whether they are reasonable and ethical, and whether the clerks are following them accurately seems to be an impossible task for a patient who questions an item on a bill.

If patients can't figure out the bills, and if employees at the facility that provides the services can't figure out the bills either, then how do the patients know if the bills are accurate or if patients are getting ripped off? What can patients do in order to ensure that they are not being cheated by billing errors? What recourses do patients have for settling disputes?

I don't have answers. My suggestion, based on my own personal experiences, is for patients to look at every piece of information that they receive from care providers and from insurance companies, and take a closer look at any items that don't seem right. Make sure that the dates match the procedure, that the procedure being billed is the right one, that the providers listed actually performed the services listed, and that the medical provider and the insurance company are talking about the same thing with the same patient's share of the cost (even if the terminology and the method of assigning categories to items are different).

Keep in mind that different facilities have different methods of handling bills with a small net amount owed by patients. Some have a policy to automatically write off amounts below a specific dollar amount, in which case the provider's bill will not match the insurance company's records, while other facilities might be quick to send the same small bills to collection agencies.

Personal Anecdote

Being off work for an extended period of time while medical bills pile up can create financial hardships on patients and their families. I had no income, and my wife's income was insufficient to cover our family's normal living expenses plus my medical bills. I did have health insurance, but my share of medical costs was more than our budget could handle. I sought help through the state's Medicaid program. This is a means-tested program. In my case, because I had health insurance, Medicaid became a supplemental policy for covering expenses after my primary insurer paid its share. Benefits begin after meeting a "paydown" amount determined by a formula. Because you don't qualify until after you have already incurred expenses, recent expenses count towards the paydown, but there is paperwork involved. I had to submit Medicaid claims against every medical billing within the relevant time period. If the expense has been paid, then the payment is credited towards the paydown amount that patients must meet before receiving benefits from Medicaid. This is a routine paperwork procedure. But one provider found a way to use this procedure to milk me for more money. They found billings which been closed because the primary insurance company had paid them according to the agreement between the care facility and the insurance company, reopened them, posted the insurance payment against the total bill, and left the amount of the negotiated discount as an open receivable - to be paid by me. My group plan (primary insurance) was typical in that each procedure had a negotiated rate of payment, and the provider agreed to only accept that amount. So when the insurance company had paid the negotiated rate, the billing was paid in full. But by reopening the billing after the fact, knowing that Medicaid was not a party to the negotiated discount rate, the amount paid by the insurance company became only a partial payment, rather than a full payment. I ended up getting hit with higher bills for past procedures solely because I needed assistance with these bills.

Only one provider used this method to create a higher payment rate for itself. I can only assume that this was done deliberately. I don't know if it was legal or not, but it is at least a very questionable billing practice from an ethical standpoint.

Personal Anecdote

Following surgery to remove a portion of my stomach, doctors and nurses were concerned because my vital signs were not stable. They were at a loss to determine a cause for this problem. There were occasions when a team of doctors from different areas of specialty would meet in my room to discuss possible causes for this problem. I wasn't a party to these conversations. I was not asked, nor would I expect to be asked, for permission for such conversations to take place. I was a very sick patient lying in a hospital bed.

As a result of decisions made during these conversations, I was transferred to various departments around the hospital for observation and numerous tests. No source of the problem was ever found, but they did manage to eliminate a number of possibilities. Eventually, the doctors were satisfied that my vitals were stable enough for me to go home, even without a known source for the problems. My hospital stay was for two weeks, which was a combination of normal recovery from a gastrectomy and testing for this unknown complication.

When the medical bills came in for services relating to this hospital visit, they included various charges relating to these in-room conferences among doctors. There were charges for "office visits". There were charges for "consultation".

I'm not going to question these specialists for deciding to bill for their time and expertise. But apparently there is no billing code designed to cover such gatherings of doctors. I could hardly consent to an "office visit" when I could barely move at all and had not been informed that such conferences would occur. At least the doctors got compensated for their time by calling this an "office visit", although I'm not sure what the going rate should be. They didn't have to employ their staff, use any office equipment or utilities, or set aside time for an appointment. As far as I can tell, they agreed to meet during their normal rounds in the hospital.

The insurance company didn't question the charges for office visits. But they refused to pay for the charges labeled "consultation". The insurance company had a specific definition of what a consultation is, and it wasn't covered under my plan.

According to the insurance company, a "consultation" is when a patient chooses to meet with a doctor in order to discuss a possible elective procedure. That isn't even remotely what happened in my case. I didn't "choose" anything. I didn't even consent to anything, because I wasn't in any condition to consent. My doctor simply decided, without my knowledge or consent because I was too sick to make such decisions, that having specialists from different areas discuss my symptoms was in my best interest. There were no consultations in terms of how the insurance company defines the term.

I discovered this after the fact, when I looked over the details of the hospital bill. It was up to me to discover this problem; it was up to me to research it; and it was up to me to follow up until the problem was corrected. I had to get the hospital to resubmit the bill to the insurance company, with these charges coded as something which the insurance company would be willing to accept. Otherwise, I would have had to pay for 100% of these charges, with no discount for group rates.

And of course, outsourced coding clerks were blamed for this problem.

Personal Anecdote

I recommend that every medical patient review their paperwork for questionable billing practices. Here is one that I missed, and it involves a large dollar amount. Following an outpatient procedure which ended up being more complicated than expected, I was required to spend a night in the hospital for observation. I was released the following morning.

In reviewing my paperwork for this book, I noticed that the hospital had billed $67,448.77 for the room. This amount was for one overnight stay for observation. How could a hospital room cost that much? The insurance company paid $11,929.82 of this amount; I paid $3,522.39. The bulk of it, $51,996.56, was written off as a negotiated discount between the provider and the insurance company. Otherwise, the paperwork sailed through with no corrections or adjustments.

I should have paid closer attention to my paperwork this at the time, but I didn't. I probably wouldn't have been able to change anything, but I would have noticed the questionable billing. I had accepted the $3,522.39 charge as being legitimate, and it might have been legitimate. But $67,448.77 for a hospital room for one night? If I had not had health insurance coverage, I would have been billed for the entire amount, $67,448.77. Uninsured patients do not get the benefit of negotiated discount prices.

Personal Anecdote

Some medical facilities make no direct effort to collect bills which are past due. Once a bill is determined to be past due, it goes directly to a collection agency. This policy is an administrative decision. Instead of paying employees to try to collect bills, they outsource the process. I should add that the entire process gets outsourced, not just the bills they have tried but failed to collect. The facility has billed the insurance company. Once the insurance company has processed the claim, then the medical facility sends out one computer-generated statement to the patient for the remaining balance. This is often done through an out of state billing company. If the bill isn't paid in full within a specified number of days, then it is sent to a collection agency. No attempt to collect is ever made by employees of the facility itself.

The problem is that in such a system, the patient sometimes doesn't get a chance to pay a bill before it goes into collection. Sometimes, the insurance company will delay processing the claim for some reason. Perhaps they need to research the validity of the claim. Often, the patient will receive a statement saying "This is not a bill. You may owe a balance after the insurance company processes the claim". Once the claim is processed by the insurance company, a computer-generated statement is sent to the patient. But if enough time has passed between the date of service and the date that the insurance company processes the claim, the bill has already been sent to a collection agency before the patient sees it.

This has happened to me on a few occasions. When it does, I refuse to recognize the collection agency a part of the process. As long as my intentions have always been to pay the bill, then I will pay the provider directly, bypassing the collection agency. If enough patients would do this, perhaps some medical facilities would think twice about their system of automatically sending bills to a collection agency before giving the patient a chance to pay. In the meantime, if the collection agency phones me about payment, I tell them that I have a legal right to insist that they no longer contact me – which I do, at least in my state. I don't know what the law says in other states.

How Do I Find the Right Doctor?

This is a serious question for me, and I doubt if I am the only one who has a problem with this. It seems to me that many people are full of advice that sounds pretty straightforward in theory. If I have concerns about my health, I get "you need to see a doctor". That makes sense, and it is sound advice that I cannot argue with. My specific problem might also give me "you need to see a specialist". I even get "my doctor is great, you need to see my doctor". If I have any problems with a medical outcome after being treated or at least diagnosed, I get "you need a second opinion" or "you need to see a different doctor in that specialty". If I don't have the strength to research what is going on with my medical treatment, I get "you need to assign a family member or somebody else to advocate for you".

This is all sound advice. I even give the same type of advice throughout this book. What to do, at least in theory, is simple. But in practice, I have to deal with the problem of how to do it. "What", I understand. "How", that is a different question. And I do not have the answer to this question.

What do you do when the only medical clinic in town tells you that you cannot see the doctor you requested because "he isn't taking new patients at this time", even though for years you have listed that doctor as your family doctor, and he does indeed see the rest of your family, yet you haven't needed his services recently and he doesn't list you as a current patient? What do you do when this same medical clinic assigns a primary care doctor to you because, out of the many doctors who serve this clinic, only one is taking on new patients? What do you do when you don't think the doctor assigned to you by the clinic is the right doctor for you, but the only clinic in town won't let you switch doctors? What do you do when you have a medical condition requiring a specialist, but your primary care doctor doesn't know enough about the condition to refer you to the correct specialty? What do you do when simply finding a different clinic in a different city isn't a practical solution? What do you do when a specialist tells you that you need tests from a different type of specialist, but you have to have a referral from your primary care physician – and the family doctor who has been assigned to you tells you that doctors in the specialty you need tests from are quacks? What do you do when you are assigned a primary care doctor who has a habit of contradicting what your specialists are advising you to do? What do you do when you have an extensive history with numerous medical specialists all working within the same network, but when a specialist tells you that you need surgery, you have no choice of surgeons – you will be referred to the same one whose previous work on you has left you seeking a second opinion? What do you do when you cannot afford to hire a medical advocate, and you don't have any family members or close friends who are able and willing to take this responsibility? What happens when your doctor has procedures in place which turn the simple task of making an appointment something to dread?

All of these questions come from my personal experiences. Given the types of problems that I encounter with finding the right doctor, how is it possible to ever get a second opinion that isn't biased towards the first opinion? I mean, what process is available to me for receiving a second opinion? My experience makes it obvious that I cannot simply walk into a different doctor's office and be checked out by a doctor who will look at my situation with fresh eyes, unbiased by conclusions drawn by other doctors. How could this lead to an unbiased second opinion? Perhaps the first doctor has misread a symptom or something, and has failed to look in the correct area for the problem. If I get a second opinion from a doctor who does not know what the first opinion was, wouldn't that make it much more likely that the same mistake in diagnosis won't be made?

I don't have answers to any of these problems. I do believe, very strongly, that we need to change the system so that individual patients have more control over which doctors they can see. Medical clinics should not be able to limit our choices.

Personal Anecdote

Before I started having health problems, I didn't really have a doctor designated as my primary care physician. My wife had one, and my daughter had the same one. Whenever I needed to list a primary care physician on a medical form, I always listed the family doctor used by the other members of my family. I had seen him occasionally, but I had never visited him often enough for him to list me as one of his patients. If I got sick, I would ask for him; but if he wasn't available, I would ask for whichever doctor at the clinic happened to be on call that day.

When I had problems with leg pain, I visited the doctor on call. When complications developed, I decided to continue with the doctor who already knew my condition. Later, when I was released from the care of the general surgeon who performed my gastrectomy, into the care of a primary physician, I requested the same doctor my wife and daughter use, the one I had always listed as my family doctor. I was told that I couldn't have the same doctor because "he isn't taking new patients now". I listed him as my doctor; he didn't list me as his patient. I was also informed that I didn't have any choice, because only one doctor at the clinic was taking new patients. I was assigned to that doctor, who by coincidence happened to be the same doctor who was on call in the emergency room whenever I went in for bleeding ulcers. At least he knew about my case, so at the time I thought he might be a good choice.

Over time, I decided that my assigned primary care physician wasn't a good match for me. He was hesitant, he didn't seem to understand anything about my specific conditions, and therefore he had difficulty finding the correct specialists to refer me to. He contradicted the orders from my surgeon. He made a point to disagree with the recommendation of a specialist even though he didn't have knowledge of the circumstances behind the recommendation.

But what could I do? I live in a rural area, and the clinic told me that this specific doctor would be my assigned doctor. It wasn't practical for me to look for a doctor in a different city.

Personal Anecdote

The local clinic wouldn't allow me to change primary care physicians. They told me who my doctor would be, and I had no choice. But I finally found a way to switch from a doctor I had little faith in. I found a smaller clinic with a new doctor who was building up a client base. I asked for an appointment.

But getting a doctor at this clinic turned out to be more complicated than simply making an appointment, even though the doctor admittedly was looking for more patients. I had to go through an application process in order to get the doctor to accept me as a patient. I had to interview for the "job" of becoming a medical patient. My records were checked. The person who processed the application discussed everything with the doctor. Finally, I received a phone call congratulating me on being accepted as a patient.

Being accepted as a patient was one thing. Getting an appointment to see the doctor was something else. In order to get an appointment, I had to talk to one specific person who was a designated scheduler. In all of the times I have called her, there has never been a time when my phone call was answered. I always have to leave a message on voicemail. When my call is returned, it is like going through the application process all over again – every single time. I can't simply state my name and reason for wanting to see my doctor. I always get grilled with question after question as if they are trying to avoid as many appointments as possible. They make me feel guilty for requesting a visit with my doctor.

I have no way around this process. There have been numerous times when I have called regarding medication and other questions which can be answered through a series of phone calls. But I have visited my doctor only one time in over two years. During that one visit, the doctor indicated a lack of knowledge regarding my specific medical problems, and I was left to rely on my specialists.

Whenever I can, I take my medical questions directly to my specialists. I feel as if I am making decisions which belong to a primary care physician. But how am I supposed to find a better way?

Don't Be Fooled by Outward Appearances

If you were facing a serious crisis in life, how would you feel if strangers constantly came up to you and made it a point to mention the problems that you are dealing with? Please, please, please everyone – unless you know a person well enough to know what he or she has been going through, do NOT make a comment about their weight. Maybe you have spent a lifetime trying to keep your weight down, but that does not mean that it is okay to tell people you barely know that they are "lucky" that they don't have your problem to deal with. If you know somebody, but you don't know them well enough to know what they are going through, don't tell them how they "look so much better" because of a change in weight. A gain in weight or a loss in weight can very well be a symptom of a serious medical condition – even if you think the person looks better or healthier with the change.

Please do not complement somebody on their "healthy" appearance unless you know them well enough to be familiar with their medical history. What you might think is a complement could very well be a painful reminder of a serious problem that somebody is dealing with.

If you have been trying to change your appearance, such as through diet and exercise, in order to receive complements from strangers, then sorry, your need for such superficial affirmation does not trump the needs of those who can be hurt by well-meaning but inappropriate comments about their outward appearance. You should be happy with how your changes have made you feel about yourself. Perhaps it is okay for you to expect family members and close friends to notice and complement you on how you have improved yourself, but I have a problem with your insensitive narcissism if you expect strangers to give you complements.

If you see somebody who looks healthy according to outward appearances, don't criticize them if they use parking spaces reserved for handicapped individuals, if they receive disability benefits, or if they receive public assistance. Don't be fooled by outward appearances. Unless you have an extensive knowledge of what these people are going through, your judgment can be extremely insensitive – and wrong.

Personal Anecdote

When I was 15 years old, my high school basketball coach listed me as 6'1" and 145 pounds. I have always been little more than skin and bones. My high school basketball teammates hated to go up against me during practices; not because I was a good player, but because they didn't like my sharp elbows. I wanted to beef up. My coach wanted me to beef up. I went into weight training. I put myself on a diet designed to build up weight. Nothing I tried actually worked.

Up until a few weeks before my gastrectomy, at age 49, my weight had never gone as high as 150 pounds. I stayed right at 145 pounds since I was 15. I never considered this to be my ideal weight. But that is the weight nature gave me.

Over all those years, I had to deal with many people who expressed jealousy over the fact that I never had to worry about being overweight. Some of these people were indeed overweight, but many of them were not. They just wanted to be thinner. I wished I had their weight problem, not my weight problem. I never considered my weight to be healthy, and I don't remember any medical professionals telling me that my weight was ideal.

I also didn't necessarily feel healthy. I had frequent heartburn, and learned that certain foods must be avoided. I had no doctor tell me which foods to avoid; I was told to figure it out by trial and error. At one point in time, during the early 1980s, I suffered from heartburn and nausea to the extent that I worried that I might have developed stomach ulcers. I went to see a doctor, one who had been recommended for me. The doctor looked at me, ran no tests and asked few questions, and told me flat out that I did not have stomach ulcers. He told me to limit my diet to foods which didn't cause heartburn. When I asked him if he had a diet plan for my situation, he said that none existed. "Just stay away from foods which cause heartburn."

Following that one visit with a doctor, my condition flared up many times. Sometimes I could equate the problem with specific foods, sometimes I couldn't. There was no diet plan for me to follow. I searched bookstores and other sources, looking through diet-related books. Regardless of what year or what decade it was, I could always find tons of books aimed at people who wanted to lose weight (whether they needed to or not). I could find absolutely no books which would help me with my particular problem.

This selection of books mirrored what goes on in society. It seemed as if everybody I met was jealous because I didn't have their weight problem. They were being fooled by outward appearances. I can't help but wonder how many of them were making themselves less healthy because they assumed that thinner was always better. Perhaps the inability of a doctor to help me, combined with a lack of published work on the subject, is symptomatic of the same reasons people develop eating disorders.

At age 49, I topped 150 pounds on the scale for the first time in my life. I made it to 155, and I thought I was on my way to a healthier body and healthier look. Within weeks, I nearly died from previously-undiagnosed bleeding ulcers.

Personal Anecdote

Throughout my adult life, my body weight had remained at about 145 pounds. It never varied until just before I had a gastrectomy, when it topped out at 155 pounds. Immediately following surgery, my body filled with fluid and the scale read 175 pounds. The fluid was removed via a thoracotomy, and my weight was down below 145 pounds. From that point on, I have not maintained the seemingly equilibrium weight that I had for the previous 40 years or so.

My weight fell when I developed new symptoms and complications from procedures. At one point in time, I was admitted to intensive care weighing only 95 pounds. I had to fight in order to get my weight back up to something which would sustain my life.

Once I regained weight, I didn't stop until I reached 185 to 190 pounds. This is about 40 pounds higher than I had ever weighed prior to my health problems. My body has finally filled out, but this is not because I am healthier. All of the health issues that I am currently experiencing, as described in this book, go along with the extra weight that I am carrying. My gastroenterologist watched me gain this weight, and told me it wasn't healthy. He told me that the weight gain is a primary cause of the acid reflux problems that continue to get worse. He told me that I had been gaining weight much too quickly, and that I should stop when my weight reached 170 pounds. But I didn't stop at 170. I have stabilized at a "new normal" weight of 185 to 190. My doctor tells me this is too much weight for someone with my health issues.

Yet everybody I meet sees me with what appears to them to be a healthier weight than they have ever seen me carry. They tell me that I must be healthier and that I must feel much better. But they are being fooled by outward appearances. I am not healthier. I do not feel better. My doctor knows it, and I know it. But people I meet in public, including longtime friends, don't understand.

Summary

I have written this book from the standpoint of a "typical" medical patient. At the beginning, I mentioned that my purpose in writing this book is to send messages to medical professionals and to other patients.

Along the way, I have included several anecdotal stories from my personal experience. Many of these stories can be classified as "horror" stories. This is by design. They are my stories, and I consider them to be horror stories.

While I have included some stories about how I considered my treatment by healthcare professionals to be very good, the majority of my stories are of the negative variety. This is not by design, but by necessity. Negative experiences stand out. Positive experiences are things that typically go unnoticed, unless they are of the "above and beyond" variety. We expect things to proceed smoothly; we notice when they don't. We can learn lessons from both positive and negative experiences.

More can and should be done to decrease negative experiences throughout the healthcare industry. Patients need to be aware that doctors are human. Medical professionals need to understand that they deal with real people and not statistics.

I consider some of my doctors to be great doctors. These great doctors are also responsible for some of the horror stories that I have included in this book. Nobody is perfect. Everybody has room for improvement.

Even great doctors make mistakes.

Appendix A: Personal Medical History

Throughout this book, I have used incidents from my personal medical history as anecdotal examples of the points that I am trying to make. My experience with the medical profession is rather extensive. Some of these stories may seem to be horrific, and in many cases that is the impression that I am trying to get across to readers.

In order to put these stories into perspective, I am including an overview of my medical history. I want to make it clear that in doing so, I am not attempting to generate sympathy for my personal situation. I am not trying to leave the impression that I consider my situation to be worse than that of many others. It would be missing the point for anybody to read my story and then say something along the lines of "I can top that". I already know that many people are going through much worse than I have gone through. I count my blessings that I am still alive; that I have the ability to physically take care of my basic needs; that I do not rely on others for constant care; that my mental capacity is as strong as it has ever been; and that I still have all my limbs and all 5 senses.

The most difficult part of writing this book has been trying to figure out how to get my points across without making it sound like I feel sorry for myself due to my personal problems, or perhaps due to the negative experiences that I have had with the medical profession. I honestly do not know the best way to emphasize this point. I hope that putting this summary of my medical history in the appendix section instead of including it as a chapter in the main section of the book will help.

*****

Most of the personal anecdotes in this book are stories relating to my current medical condition, so I will begin this summary of my medical condition at the point in time when I first began to seek medical help for conditions that I am currently dealing with.

2004-2005

I had a stent implant on October 1, 2004 for a closed artery in my right leg. Complications included drop-foot, which required extensive rehab involving a foot specialist, an orthotic brace, and a physical therapist.

My first indication that something might be wrong came when I couldn't walk through my yard without turning my ankle on the uneven ground. When I mowed the lawn, I kept stepping in little holes in the yard, and my ankle would end up in unnatural positions. I had experience with ankle sprains during my days as a basketball player, and I know what they look like. This was different. My ankle would turn completely sideways, on several occasions, yet there never was any pain or swelling in the area of my ankle. I knew something wasn't quite right.

There was another kind of pain associated with this. My right leg would hurt whenever I walked. The pain seemed to start in the upper thigh area and move downward. The pain would go away after I would sit down to rest. I would have to rest several times before I could finish mowing the lawn.

This pain-while-walking occurred at other times, not just while I was mowing the lawn. For example, I couldn't walk through a store without being forced by pain to stop and rest in the middle of an aisle.

I knew something was wrong, so I went to see a doctor. I had no pulse in my ankle and no feeling in my right foot. The reaction from the doctor, a general practitioner, was along the lines of "Oh my God, I hope we caught this in time. Otherwise, you'll get gangrene and lose your leg!" I was referred to a vascular surgeon.

Thankfully, the specialist did not echo the fatalistic expression of the general practitioner. I was given an angiogram, and it was discovered that I had a blocked artery in my right leg. For this, I received a stent implant which reopened the artery.

Unfortunately, I did experience some complications. I developed drop foot (or foot drop). My right foot would not move properly when I walked, and I had to drag it behind. I was referred to a neurologist. My drop foot was eventually cured, but only after extensive rehab which involved an orthotic brace and physical therapy.

I also frequently get painful callouses on the bottom of my feet. I can get relief from this pain by shaving off these callouses. They reappear, so the pain relief is always temporary. This problem continues to this day. My physical therapist advised me to switch to a specific shoe brand and wear a larger shoe. I now wear shoes that are two full sizes larger than before.

2006

This one was a biggie, a life-changer. It was my first near-death experience, and I continue to have health problems related to this incident.

It started one morning while I was driving to work. All of a sudden, it felt as if my entire chest and abdominal cavities were attacking me. I really can't explain what this sensation felt like, but something was definitely wrong – something which I had never before experienced. I had to pull the car over and stop, even though at the time I was only a few feet away from the parking lot at work. I sat there for several minutes, not being able to move. I wasn't sure if the sensation would ever end or if I was going to die right then. Eventually, the worst of it ended. But I knew something still wasn't right. I was weak and dizzy. The only thing I could think about was that I had to get to a doctor. Even though I was only a few feet from work, I didn't go to work. I was afraid that I would pass out while trying to walk up the steps to get there – and that I might die if I passed out. I drove back home, called into work to let them know I was going to be out sick that day, and then I went to see a doctor.

When I checked in at the doctor's office, I had to fill out routine paperwork explaining the health complaint which prompted me to request a doctor, my symptoms, and a detailed checklist involving my medical history. For some reason which I do not understand, the doctor focused entirely on one item on that checklist – an incident that occurred more than 40 years earlier when I was 9 years old. In 1966, I had been hospitalized for what I understand to be a blocked colon.

Was there a connection between my symptoms on that day in 2006 and the 1966 incident? I don't know. I certainly have had my share of colon problems since 2006. The doctor prescribed medication. I don't remember what the medication was, but based on what I have learned since then it must have acted as a blood thinner.

That night, I nearly bled to death. I had a sudden need for a bowel movement, or so I thought. What I passed was blood, and lots of it. I was weak and barely conscious. Blood was all over the bathroom floor. When I finally tried to move, I fell down in the hallway and left another pile of blood to be cleaned up. From there, I could not move. I had to just lay there and wait for the ambulance to arrive. My wife had called the ambulance for me.

I was given blood in the emergency room. I was going in and out of consciousness, and the emergency room doctor kept yelling in my face to "stay with us". He later told me that he hadn't expected me to survive the night. He tried in vain to call in a surgeon to perform an emergency surgery. Apparently, only one surgeon was on duty at my rural hospital, and he was busy performing surgery at a nearby rural hospital. He wasn't available, so I was flown by helicopter to an urban hospital.

I had an emergency partial gastrectomy for bleeding ulcers. They didn't remove all of my stomach, but they got a large chunk of it. They didn't remove all of the ulcers. They did remove one which the surgeon told me was the size of a grapefruit.

All told, I had been given 24 units of blood by the time the surgery was over. Nurses on my floor in the hospital kept referring to me as "the guy who took 24 units of blood". None of the nurses had experience with a patient who had been given so much blood in such a short period of time. They were surprised that I could go through that and still be alive.

Immediately following surgery, I developed complications. My vital signs would not stabilize. My chest cavity filled with fluid, and I had a thoracotomy to remove fluid from around my lungs. The fluid had caused even my extremities to appear bloated. What seemed to worry the hospital staff the most was the tendency of my blood pressure to reach levels which were dangerously low. I remained in the hospital for two weeks while doctors tried to figure out what was wrong. Doctors from different specialties visited me. These different specialists huddled together in my room and speculated about what the problem might be. I was transferred to various areas in the hospital for testing and monitoring. They never did figure out what the problem was. After two weeks, I was told that my vital signs had stabilized enough for me to go home. At the time of my release from the hospital, I asked the nurse if I should continue to take the medicine which had been prescribed for me by the family doctor when I first experienced symptoms. Since this medication wasn't mentioned in the paperwork accompanying my release, the nurse checked with the surgeon. The answer I got was "definitely not, that medicine almost killed you when it caused your bleeding". They didn't put that diagnosis in writing, but that is what I was told.

I didn't feel any better after I was able to go home from the hospital. I was weak, the incision area was painful and herniated, and I was nauseated. I vomited frequently. After a couple of follow-up appointments with the surgeon, I was released to return to work. I was still very sick, and they had never found the source of my complications. But I was released for work anyway, because "the book" on a gastrectomy says that I was recovered. The surgeon said that he had to go by the book, and there wasn't anything else he could do. When I returned to work, my supervisor saw how sick I was and sent me home with instructions to not come back until I was better. I took those instructions to the primary care physician who had recently been assigned to me by the local medical clinic. He agreed to give me a few more weeks to recover at home. After that, I returned to work. But I was still sick from unknown causes.

2007-2008

My recovery from stomach surgery never proceeded according to expectations. I was living with nausea and cramping on a daily basis. I was weak. I had constant, unbearable pain. I fought through it, and continued to try to keep my job. Every day was a long nightmare for me. Normal activities which I had always taken for granted became stressful events. I associated the new-found stress with incidents of cramping, so I switched to a different job which I considered to be less stressful. This attempt at job-switching failed, and I had no choice but to quit my job. When I did so, I applied for Social Security Disability benefits, a process that literally takes years to go through.

I also had no answers as to why this was happening to me. I continued to undergo medical tests in an attempt to find out what was wrong. Following one upper GI, the gastroenterologist personally phoned me with the results. He told me I had "big problems", that I would have to live with them for the rest of my life, and that there was medication which would help to alleviate the problem but not fix it entirely. He told me that my esophagus had deteriorated into "hamburger". This diagnosis was devastating, and I was thankful that the doctor delivered it to me in a professional and compassionate manner. I was in pain, I had just received bad news about my health, but the doctor who gave me the bad news earned my respect for the way he handled the situation.

This diagnosis explained some of the problems I was going through. It explained my acid reflux, for example. But it did not explain all of my pains, cramping, nausea, etc. I continued to have more scopes in an attempt to find the source of my other problems and also as a follow-up for esophagitis. Abnormal polyps were removed, and in at least one instance sent to a nationally-recognized expert for diagnosis. At one point in time, the results were labeled as "pre-cancerous". This meant, among other things, that I would be undergoing more frequent upper and lower scopes.

While I was going through all of this, I made one final attempt to hold down a job. I knew I couldn't go back to the same type of work that I did before. I found a job which involved little physical exertion in a relatively stress-free environment. The pay was less than I had become accustomed to, but it was a job.

Meanwhile, I was still searching for answers to ongoing health problems.

2009-2010

I had another stent implant similar to the one in 2004. I was told that it is not abnormal for a new stent to be required after 5 years. I was told that this one was more complicated than the first one, and I was required to stay overnight for observations following this outpatient procedure.

I had never recovered as expected following the gastrectomy in 2006. In fact, my symptoms continued to worsen. I reached the point where I spent an average of about four days per week vomiting. On the days when I wasn't vomiting, I would feel weak and dizzy - as if I was about to pass out. I was forced to give up on my final attempt to hold down some kind of job.

I had no medical explanation for this, so the doctors continued to schedule tests. Eventually I was diagnosed as having had a stroke in my colon, with the 2006 surgery considered to be the most likely time frame. I underwent a reversible colostomy in March of 2010. I needed assistance from home-care nurses following this procedure.

Complications arose immediately. The colostomy bag did not work as expected. I was given Hegar dilators in an attempt to correct for this problem, but they only created excruciating pain. I couldn't use them without causing this pain, and neither could the home nurses. Several different nurses tried in vain. When the surgeon saw first-hand what I was going through, during a follow-up medical visit, he immediately stopped all attempts. I went directly from the doctor's office to the hospital for an early colostomy reversal surgery.

Following this surgery, the pain and nausea persisted, and I began losing weight. Within a month, I was back in the emergency room. The emergency room doctor did nothing for me, other than to call in a priest to read my last rights. It took my family members to convince this doctor that if he wasn't able to do anything for me, I should be transferred to the hospital where my recent surgeries had taken place. Another life-flight helicopter ambulance ride took me to that hospital. I spent a day or so in the intensive care unit before I was transferred to a regular hospital room. I weighed 95 pounds at the time. I was extremely weak, I could barely eat, and I didn't really understand what was happening to me at the time. My paperwork says things like "abdominal abscess with follow-up sonograms" and "interventional radiology". I know I was told it had something to do with infection. My food intake was monitored, and I was required to remain hospitalized until the doctor was satisfied that my calorie and protein intake increased to a sufficient level. I was being told to eat the same foods which happened to be my favorites, yet I had a very difficult time doing so. To remove fluid buildup around the infected area near the surgery incision in my abdomen from the previous colon surgeries, I underwent a procedure called abscess incision and drainage. The drainage is known as Jackson Pratt Drain Care. This was a drainage tube inserted in my abdomen. Now, in place of a colostomy bag which had only recently been removed, I had a drainage tube with a cup that I had to empty after documenting the volume of discharge. Over the course of several weeks, I had numerous follow-up outpatient procedures associated with this JP Drain. Also, I was required to have home care nurses return to help monitor my output as well as my food intake.

2011-2015

I began experiencing blood loss. I didn't know I was losing blood until March of 2011, when a routine blood test preceding another angiogram for my leg pain indicated that I had extreme anemia. The angiogram was cancelled and I was immediately admitted to the hospital. I was in the hospital for a few days, and during that time I received blood transfusions. I also received a colonoscopy for the purpose of determining the source of the bleeding. The bleeding did occur in the colon area, but it was never determined what caused the bleeding. I battled anemia for the next two years or more. I had multiple blood transfusions and regularly-scheduled blood tests during this time frame. In 2013 I had a wireless capsule enteroscopy, which involved swallowing a pill with a camera to look for abnormalities and a source of bleeding. The procedure did not reveal the source of bleeding, but eventually I got the bleeding under control through medication. I still don't know why I had been experiencing blood loss. During this time frame, I continued to get frequent colonoscopy and upper-GI scopes. A typical clinical report following these scopes would list the following: Barrett's Esophagus, Gastrointestinal Bleeding and Iron Deficiency Anemia.

My first attempt at an angiogram for possible stenting in 2011 failed in March because the blood test revealed anemia. My second attempt failed in August because of chest pains. I had recently started experiencing chest pains, and I mentioned it when I was admitted for the angiogram. I was already prepped for the procedure when the vascular surgeon came into the room and learned about the chest pains. He arranged for me to be transferred to the heart unit of the hospital, where I underwent the angiogram for my heart instead of for my leg pain. The speculation was that I had experienced one or more heart attacks, and they made arrangements for possible heart surgery. Luckily, I didn't need heart surgery. The procedure revealed a healthy heart, but it also revealed a previously-undetected artery blockage near the aorta. This required no corrective medical procedure, however, because it had already self-corrected by developing a natural bypass. ("100% stenosis in the Proximal right coronary artery 20 mm long and 2 mm in diameter - distal vessel fills via collaterals from the Circumflex", according to my paperwork). I was prescribed heart medication, but it was later determined that my chest pains were symptoms of esophagitis and were not heart-related. A diligent cardiovascular surgeon, poring over my medical records, suspected that the esophagus and not the heart was the source of these chest pains. A nuclear cardiac stress test confirmed the suspicions. The doctor told me that this was due to esophagitis; the terminology used in my paperwork is "acute peptic ulcer with hemorrhage". I still experience these chest pains, but they are less frequent. Knowing the source of the pains allows me to treat them with the proper medication.

I was able to go through with the planned angiogram for my leg pain on the third attempt, in June 2012. However, the only blockage which was found, and which is presumed to be the source of the pain, was in an area which cannot be fixed through stenting. The vascular surgeon showed sincere concern for my pain. I was offered medication to treat it, something he calls walking pills, but the medication had side effects worse than the leg pain. I chose not to continue with this medication. The same doctor scheduled an abdominal ultrasound in case it would reveal a problem and a source of my leg pain which an angiogram could not detect. The results of that procedure were negative. The leg pains are not getting worse over time, and they are not expected to get worse. I will continue to follow up with my specialist to make sure that it doesn't get worse.

Most of the problems I dealt with in this time frame are ongoing problems relating to complications from surgery, pain, acid reflux, weakness, nausea, and bleeding. Some of these areas of concern are problems which I have been told cannot be corrected. I have to deal with these issues the best I can through medication. Other areas, however, remain unexplained. These continue to be concerns for which I am trying to find medical explanations, and hopefully, these explanations will lead to corrective measures. Even if these problems cannot be corrected, I need to know what is causing them and why I have to live with the pain. Appendix B includes more details on these ongoing concerns.

Appendix B: Pain Controls My Life, but Doctors Don't Want To Treat It or Discuss It

I have not had a pain-free moment for ten years. Unless you count the times I am asleep – but pain has drastically disrupted my sleeping patterns. I often fall asleep out of sheer exhaustion after pain has prevented me from falling asleep when I know I need to. My pain is all-consuming.

I'm not talking about chronic pain from a single source. I think I can relate to people who go through that type of problem. But the type of pain I have is something entirely different. I have multiple sources of pain. At any given point in time, one source of pain is likely to be dominant over all other sources of pain. This doesn't mean that the other pains have gone away; it just means that they are somewhat hidden behind a more dominant pain. Eventually, a different pain will rise to the level of being the dominant pain. The various sources of pain take turns that way, alternating which pain is dominant. But they don't alternate because one dominant pain decreases. They alternate because the other pains increase. The trend over time is always more pain, not less pain.

*

I describe one type of pain as the sensation that there are several fish hooks stuck in my rear end. Sometimes it also seems that there are fish hooks throughout my abdominal cavity. This pain never goes away. It gets worse following every bowel movement and after I pass gas, but this pain is always present. For this, my doctor has prescribed numerous combinations of the same set of medications. According to the doctor, these medications are supposed to eliminate the source of the pain. According to the doctor, this is a quick fix for a common ailment. But after two years of using this medication; two years of making adjustments in search of a specific combination of these medications; two years of being told that I need to keep searching for just the right combination; two years of being told that the problem is simple to fix; two years of asking if perhaps there might be something else going on to cause my problem, something that requires a different treatment, and being told no, this is the approach I need to take – I have made absolutely no progress. I could understand making adjustments if the medication has shown some signs that it is having any effect at all on the source of the pain. But no such signs exist. The symptoms never change, no matter which combination of medications I try. The pain continues to gradually worsen over time. After two years, I have given up on trying new combinations of medication for this problem. I continue to take the medicine that has been prescribed, but I quit asking the doctor to prescribe a new combination. Two years has convinced me that no combination will work, and that the same doctor will not consider a different approach.

The doctor in question is the surgeon who performed my colon surgeries. He has been treating my pain as a complication from my surgeries, which I believe it is. But since I haven't been able to make progress using his approach, I asked my gastroenterologist to look into this specific problem. He listened to my complaint. I asked if there was another surgeon who could give me a second opinion on the problem and the treatment plan. I was told that there was no other surgeon in this specialty whom I could be referred to. The gastroenterologist took another look at pictures in my file from recent colonoscopies, and told me that the incision area of my colon had become ulcerated. In terms of information given to me, this was a new diagnosis from an old picture. He told me that to fix it would require another colon surgery performed by the same surgeon. I had another colonoscopy to make sure that surgery was still indicated, but it wasn't. The gastroenterologist told me that the ulcers had healed enough to make surgery unnecessary at this point in time.

To the gastroenterologist, this meant that no follow-up was necessary, other than to watch for changes during my next scheduled colonoscopy. In terms of my pain, I was back where I started, with the same questions and no answers. The healing that this latest procedure indicated had not resulted in a reduction of pain. I was left with no new treatment plan for the pain.

This is a typical outcome for medical tests and procedures which I have undergone in recent years. According to the doctor, a negative test result means that a problem doesn't exist. According to what I am living with, a negative test result means that no diagnosis has been made for a problem that I know does exist. This difference between a doctor's viewpoint on test results and my viewpoint on test results is something that I have been dealing with for several years now. Even when the doctor goes into a procedure with an understanding that the purpose of the procedure is to find answers or to eliminate possibilities, that purpose seems to get lost in the aftermath of a negative test result. The doctor treats a "good" test result as a victory; I think of it as one step in finding a source of a known problem.

This pattern gets repeated whenever my symptoms worsen. I end up with no answers.

This is similar to what I had previously gone through, for nearly four years, until doctors finally quit looking at my stomach for a source of my sickness and found out that part of my colon was dead.

This type of pain makes sitting down or lying down intolerable. It makes it nearly impossible for me to concentrate on anything except for my pain. It makes falling asleep impossible. The only way that I can reduce this pain to a more tolerable level is to stick a finger in my rear end to absorb collected moisture. This is something I do several times every single day, and again at bedtime. It isn't something that is pleasant to think about, or to do to myself. It is the only thing I have found that reduces the pain, even though the pain relief is short-lived.

*

I continue to suffer from the leg pain which first appeared more than ten years ago. I have had stent implants on two separate occasions for this. The stents worked well for a period of time, but the pain is back, probably to stay.

I have been seeing a cardiovascular surgeon who understands what I am going through, and has made some commendable efforts to alleviate the pain. He has performed an angiogram, looking for a source of the pain – a source which can be corrected through stenting. He did find a blockage which could explain my pain, but it isn't something that is correctible through stenting. He offered me some medication, what he calls "walking pills", to alleviate the pain. I tried those, but for me the side effects were worse than the pain. The leg pain goes away when I sit down to rest my leg. It hasn't been getting any worse, a potential problem that the doctor has been concerned about. As long as the pain doesn't get worse, there is no indication that this problem will lead to more problems in the future. It was my choice to reject the medication. I would rather have leg pain which I know how to control than daily headaches from medication.

I underwent an abdominal ultrasound at the suggestion of the cardiovascular surgeon. This was done in case there was a source of pain which isn't revealed through an angiogram – another attempt by the doctor to find a way to lessen my pain. The ultrasound came back negative, meaning that it didn't reveal any such source of pain. But the ultrasound process itself was very painful for me.

*

I have abdominal pain and discomfort. The ultrasound on my abdomen was painful because it involved direct pressure on my abdomen. My abdomen is painful when touched. In addition, I suffer from a lot of discomfort originating from the abdominal area. My intestines seem to be constantly active. Pressure and tightening of the abdomen are normal for me. Bloating and gas are constantly present, but they seem to get worse at night and during times when I feel stressed. Occasional cramping occurs. My abdominal pain and discomfort always gets worse during times when my acid reflux is at its worse. The upper and lower problems flare up at the same time. It seems as if the abdominal pressure, when it releases, erupts in both directions. Because of this, I suspect that a common source may exist for both my upper abdomen and lower abdomen pain and discomfort. I mentioned to my gastroenterologist that I believed these problems should be looked at together in search of a common source. I was told that these problems involve different medical specialties. As a result, nobody is looking into the possibility of a common source for my upper and lower medical issues. The same doctor performs both upper and lower scopes, and refers me to other specialists when he decides it is necessary.

*

One problem I worry about is blood loss. I have had to deal with anemia since my colon surgeries. I have had several transfusions. I have had colonoscopies for the specific purpose of looking for a source of the blood loss. I have gone through a period of time when I was required to have regular blood tests to monitor my blood count. Once, I had a wireless capsule enteroscopy, in which I swallowed a capsule with a camera to look for bleeding sources. I haven't had incidents of anemia since I began taking high doses of Asacol (4800 mg daily for 2 years and counting). The medication seems to have stopped the bleeding, but I was never given a reason why the bleeding was occurring in the first place. A colonoscopy

124

indicated that bleeding occurred in the colon, but didn't indicate why this bleeding occurred.

I was told that I would notice when I was anemic because I would feel particularly weak. But that hasn't been the case. I suffer from constant weakness. There have been times in recent months when I felt particularly weak, and worried that the increased weakness was due to anemia. In these instances, I asked for blood tests. But recent tests have indicated that my blood count is normal. I have not been able to associate any symptoms, including weakness, with anemia.

*

Acid reflux is a major concern for me. I get regular upper GI scopes because I have Barrett's Esophasus and related problems. I have been told that I will have to deal with this condition for the rest of my life. Recent results of these scopes tend to show either no worsening or a slight improvement in my condition. I started with level 4 esophagitis, and more recently I was told that it had improved to level 2 – whatever that means. But my symptoms tell me that the condition is getting worse. There have been times when I have changed the medication for this condition. Perhaps the medication becomes less effective over time and needs to be changed; perhaps not. My doctors have been trying to find the most effective medication for this condition. I get samples of new medications when they come on the market. I have several different medications available to me as options for treating these symptoms, but these medications tend to be very expensive. Medicare doesn't cover all of them.

My symptoms have gotten worse over time, but perhaps not because the medication is becoming less effective. Perhaps the symptoms involve something else, something which has yet to be diagnosed. I have noticed a strong connection between my acid reflux and symptoms relating to my intestines. Both the upper and lower areas flare up at the same time. It's like an explosion which goes in both directions. I have not been diagnosed with anything which would explain this connection, but the connection is definitely there – according to my symptoms.

Acid reflux is not the same thing as heartburn, although recently I have experienced heartburn along with acid reflux. When acid reflux flares up, I need a lot of time to recover in order to function properly. At some point almost every night, I wake up choking on reflux. It gets so bad that I feel like I could drown in it. It leaves an awful taste in my mouth. Because of the nightly problems with acid reflux, I haven't been able to sleep in a bed for several years. No matter how I arrange pillows, a bed doesn't give me the support that I get from a couch arm rest. I have to switch positions several times during the night. I cannot eliminate the problem no matter what I do. I can't remember the last time I had a full and restful night's sleep.

My problem with reflux isn't limited to nights or times when I am trying to sleep. It is noticeably worse at night, but that isn't the only time it occurs. I get it during the day on most days.

Acid reflux also can take the form of severe chest pains. Whether choking on it, or suffering chest pains, it always feels like it settles in the back of my brain, near the top of my spinal cord. I am always unable to function properly following these incidents. It is normal for me to be unable to do anything productive for a full day following a single incident. On many days, I don't have the energy to get dressed.

*

On good days, I am lucky if I can manage to have an hour or two of total productive time. I can do so much, and then I just can't go on any longer. When I get up in the morning, on my good days, I never know for sure how long or exactly which part of the day I will be productive. I do what I can, and when the sensation hits, the rest of my day is shot. This is difficult to explain, but the accompanying sensation tells me that this problem is directly related to the reflux or my esophagitis.

I spend most of my time at home. I have to travel out of town for my medical appointments, and I know ahead of time that when I have to go out of town, I will be incapacitated the next day for the full day. I have to plan around that inevitability. On occasion, I have had two such appointments in the same week. When that happens it takes an additional toll. I might be down for almost all of the following week. On rare occasions, I go out of town just to get away for a few hours – to eat at my favorite restaurant, for example. I do that knowing full well that I will be incapacitated the next day.

My problems are worse at night. Every night - along with flare-ups of acid reflux - I get alternate hot and cold feelings. This is something which I find unbearable, and it makes me feel weaker. I end up lying down, alternating between having a fan blow cool air on me and adding layers of clothing. I have missed many of my daughter's school activities because of this. I cannot bear to sit in a crowd at night, and when I have tried I end up having to leave the room. These nighttime problems always begin shortly after the sun goes down, meaning that they start earlier during long winter nights than they do during long summer days.

I have other pains which I am not listing, because I believe they are incidental to the major problems which I am trying to focus on.

*

I would be able to accept my current medical condition if I had a diagnosis for each of my medical problems, explaining why these problems cannot be corrected. But I do not have a medical explanation for all of it. I undergo colonoscopies. I undergo upper GIs. I undergo other tests. When the tests come back negative, or at least not worse than the previous one, then I am left without answers. In the meantime, I have pain - lots of pain, from numerous sources. I haven't had a pain-free day for over ten years.

I do not take any kind of pain medication, other than regular-strength Tylenol which does nothing for my chronic pain. I only use Tylenol for incidental pains unrelated to my chronic conditions. I want to get my problems diagnosed properly, and hopefully they can be corrected so that the pain goes away. If I had been given medical reasons for all of my symptoms, then I wouldn't be searching for answers. If it turns out that there are medical reasons why my problems cannot be corrected, then I would expect my doctors to treat my pain. But in the meantime, I am in constant pain and I worry about the possibility that some pains are symptoms of a serious yet undiagnosed medical condition. When I mention pain to my doctors, they are quick to change the subject. In my experience, doctors will do anything to control a conversation with a patient in order to avoid discussing the realities of chronic pain.

It seems as if doctors want to run and hide whenever I bring up the subject of pain. Sometimes, a doctor or a nurse will ask me to give them a number between one and ten to rank my pain, as a standard question. But when I try to go into more detail about my specific pain, they quickly change the subject.

It seems as if none of my doctors has an understanding of what patients with chronic pain are going through. One doctor deflected my concerns by equating my chronic pain with his own excruciating pain from a medical procedure he had to recover from. "We all have to live with it", he told me. Then he left the room, not giving me a chance to explain that his pain was not the same thing as the chronic pain that I have suffered with for over ten years. The "rank your current pain on a scale from one to ten" question is completely irrelevant for chronic-pain sufferers. There simply is no base for comparison of numbers. When doctors or nurses ask me that question, I know that they don't understand chronic pain. I refuse to give a number when I am asked. Instead, I try to talk about the nature of my pain. But that's when the subject gets changed.

Only one doctor has seriously discussed a pain management plan with me. But no actual plan got set up. The plan that was discussed involved me learning how to live with pain, and included no steps to reduce pain. I don't need help living with pain; I need pain reduction. With this discussion, I was prescribed Tramadol as a pain reliever. Along with this prescription was a stern warning that the doctor would never prescribe anything stronger for me. I took Tramadol for a full year, as prescribed. But it never did anything at all to reduce my chronic pain. So after a year, I chose not to renew the prescription. I was getting no benefit from it.

I don't want pain medication, anyway. I think of chronic pain as a symptom of something else, and perhaps as a clue for finding an undiagnosed illness. I want the sources of the pain to be corrected. But if that cannot be done, then pain medication will be necessary. Currently, I have no doctor following up on my urgent problems. I set up an appointment for the specific purpose of discussing this lack of follow-up. I got a sympathetic ear, followed by an appointment for yet another colonoscopy. But when that scope didn't reveal the source of the problem, the same doctor failed to offer me another course of action for locating the problem. He simply noted that there was nothing new to be concerned with, and closed the book on the incident until my next scheduled colonoscopy. When my problems flared up again, I set up another appointment to discuss the same thing I had discussed before. But this time, instead of the doctor meeting with me, he had an assistant meet with me. The assistant, whom I had never met before, told me at the beginning of the conversation that because she hadn't worked on my case, she couldn't discuss the very things that I specifically made the appointment to discuss. The office visit was a complete waste of time.

*

I have smoked cigarettes throughout my adult life. I tried to quit on numerous occasions throughout the years. I have tried just about every method that has been suggested for me. The method I have tried most often is quitting cold turkey. I have tried various substitutes for holding a cigarette. I have tried different types of non-tobacco cigarettes. I have tried brand-switching. I went through a stop-smoking program administered by the local hospital, which not only involved brand switching but also peer-support. I tried nicotine gum, as well as the stop-smoking program that I received with the purchase of the gum. I have used nicotine patches; when they didn't work the first time, I went through the series of patches a second time. I tried Chantix. I was using Chantix, prescribed by my primary care physician at my request, when I entered the hospital for colon surgery. The hospital staff took me off of it while I was in the hospital. They didn't explain why they removed it from my medication, but I have learned since then that Chantix can be dangerous for people with my medical history. The only stop-smoking method that I have heard of but never tried is hypnosis, and I have never had a doctor recommend that method for me.

I am well aware of the dangers of smoking. I know what damage it does to the body of a smoker. I know what it can do to family members of a smoker. I know the financial cost of smoking. I feel the ever-increasing social pressure faced by smokers. I certainly don't enjoy being hounded about smoking. And I am aware of the dangers of smoking which are specific to my known medical conditions. Smoking is an addiction. I can say that I am physically addicted to cigarettes. It is also a psychological addiction. I am addicted to the pleasures which I associate with smoking. Whenever I am trying to quit, I have a very difficult time with the pains associated with nicotine withdrawal.

I have plenty of incentives to quit smoking. I have been unsuccessful in every previous attempt to quit, but that doesn't mean I won't keep trying. I know that many ex-smokers had made several unsuccessful attempts before they finally achieved success. I know there is always hope that the next attempt will work.

But with my present medical condition, my priorities are necessarily different. My entire life is being dictated by pain and discomfort. Every waking moment, I am in pain. I can't get a good night's sleep because of pain and discomfort. On good days, I am lucky to be able to spend an hour or two doing something productive. I can't do yard work or other physical activities. I can't go anywhere, including to the grocery store, without adding to my pain and without needing recovery time after I return home. When I push myself to do more in any given day, the following day's side effects are worse. Everyday things which I used to take for granted tend to add to my pain and discomfort. Even the process of showing up for my doctors' appointments increases the pain, and requires a full day of recovery before I can do anything productive. I simply cannot add the discomfort of nicotine withdrawal on top of everything else. My pain is already beyond my ability to cope; I certainly won't voluntarily add more pain on top of what I already have. I don't suppose that people who haven't experienced long-term situations with all-consuming pain and discomfort would understand this point. By necessity, long term problems become less significant when all I can think about is my current pain.

It would be different if it could be shown that my daily pain would be reduced if I quit smoking - in other words, if smoking was the source of my pain, and this source of pain would disappear if I didn't continue to smoke. But that is not the case. I have asked multiple doctors if my illnesses would clear up if I quit smoking. The standard answer I get is along the lines of "well, smoking doesn't help to heal you", which doesn't answer the question at all. When I respond by asking for a yes or no answer to my question, the doctors either say no or admit that they don't think so. When I ask if they could suggest a stop-smoking program which would not add more pain to my existing pain, my doctors all say no.

My pain will kill me if I can't find a way to get it under control. It is at an unsustainable level. If the pain doesn't kill me, then it will be the undiagnosed sources of the pain which will kill me. If my years of smoking turns out to be a contributing factor (which so far it hasn't, but it could), then that fact would be irrelevant to the question of how to move forward. That is in the past. Moving forward, continuing to smoke as opposed to quitting (a completely separate issue from past smoking) could shorten my life. But that will never happen if my chronic pain sources are allowed to get me first. I'm not opposed to a discussing of the need to quit smoking. I am not opposed to this discussion taking place as it relates to my current medical worries. I am opposed to the discussion taking place instead of, and out of context of, my current medical worries.

Not all of my physical problems have been successfully diagnosed. I have many unanswered questions, and they will continue to be unanswered as long as my doctors are not focused on finding answers. I have not been given a medical reason for all of my pain and discomfort. For most of these pains, I have not been told that I will have to live with them for the rest of my life. From my point of view, finding answers to these questions is the most important thing in my life right now. Yet my doctors are not looking for answers. They run the same tests over and over, and these tests do not yield answers. When I complain, they schedule more of the same tests.

Instead of focusing on my specific problems, some of my doctors tend to want to focus on my smoking habit. I understand that damage from smoking is a concern for doctors. It is a concern for me. I never back down from discussing this issue with my doctors. But a discussion of smoking is often used as a substitute for, instead of an addition to, a discussion of my current medical condition and my reason for seeing the doctor in the first place. Doctors seem to be programmed to see a smoker and not look past the smoking. I see a doctor because I have undiagnosed medical problems, and the doctor tries to take control of the conversation to make it about smoking - while completely ignoring the symptoms that I came to see him about. I see a doctor because of complications from previously diagnosed problems, or for complications from surgery, and the conversation switches from my immediate problems to the fact that I smoke. When I fill out paperwork at check-in, and check off all of the boxes that relate to my current symptoms and the reason for my visit, the doctor most likely will never comment on any of the symptoms but will notice right away that I marked "yes" for being a smoker.

I tell my doctors that I will be glad to discuss a stop-smoking program with them in the proper context of dealing with the problems at hand, which are: undiagnosed pain and discomfort; complications from surgeries which have not been declared to be permanent; complications from previously-diagnosed illnesses which are not responding to medication and treatment; and most of all, pain reduction, which I believe will come with proper diagnosis and treatment of the problems which I am seeing the doctors for. All I ask for is a reduction in pain before I consider adding the pain of nicotine withdrawal. But all too often, these problems don't get discussed. The doctors can't seem to put all of the current issues into perspective. They have tunnel vision which prevents them from looking beyond the smoking issue. I have been misdiagnosed on at least two previous occasions due to this tunnel vision – once when I had an emergency due to bleeding ulcers, and once when it was first discovered that I had circulation problems in my right leg. Now, I am having difficulty finding a doctor who will actually listen to my problems and consider all of the symptoms. I realize that doctors today are very busy, but when they decide to control the conversation, the patients' concerns get short-shafted.

I do not use alcohol or any illegal drugs.

I have seen several doctors in recent years – at least three general practitioners and many different specialists – and not one of them has indicated an understanding of what a patient with chronic pain is going through, or a willingness to discuss the issue. Every time I bring up the subject of chronic pain, my doctors quickly change the subject, and then they leave the room.

*****

*****